Burn Melt Shred

Also by Ian K. Smith, M.D.

Plant Power

Fast Burn

Mind over Weight

Clean & Lean

The Clean 20

Blast the Sugar Out!

The SHRED Power Cleanse

The SHRED Diet Cookbook

SUPER SHRED

SHRED

The Truth About Men

Eat

Happy

The 4 Day Diet

Extreme Fat Smash Diet

The Fat Smash Diet

The Take-Control Diet

Dr. Ian Smith's Guide to Medical Websites

Novels

The Ancient Nine

The Blackbird Papers

The Unspoken

Wolf Point

BURN

MELT

SHRED

Transform Your Body in 8 Weeks

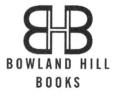

The information in this book is not intended to replace the advice of the reader's own physician or other medical professional. You should consult a medical professional in matters relating to health, especially if you have existing medical conditions, and before starting, stopping, or changing the dose of any medication you are taking. Individual readers are solely responsible for their own health care decisions. The author and the publisher do not accept responsibility for any adverse effects individuals may claim to experience, whether directly or indirectly, from the information contained in this book.

First published in the United States by Bowland Hill Books

www.DoctorIanSmith.com

ISBN 979-8-788-50006-5 (paperback)
ISBN 978-0-578-34731-8 (e-book)

First Edition: 2021

10 9 8 7 6 5 4 3 2 1

To my twin brother, Dana, who constantly reminds me what it means to be fearless and to never be afraid to strike out on your own and follow your heart.

CONTENTS

A Note from the Author

I decided to do something I've never done before. I am trying to help as many people as possible at the same time lose weight, get healthy, feel better, and learn healthier lifestyle habits. That part is not new, as I've been doing that for many years. The part that is new is that I'm self-publishing this book and making it affordable to EVERYONE.

I have spent the bulk of my career trying to reach and impact as many people as possible, regardless of age, race, religious affiliation, gender, or nationality. It's simply in my DNA to help people, and I derive a tremendous amount of pleasure doing so. Some people like flashy awards or headlines or trophies. I like people using and benefiting from some of my teachings and letting me know that in some way I have changed their life for the better. That is my oxygen as well as the fire that ignites my engine.

This book is slim, no-nonsense, and straight forward. This is by design! I don't want you spending hours reading a dense treatise on nutrition, exercise, and weight loss. I have plenty of other books you can choose in my bibliography that will fulfill that need. Instead, I want you to spend your precious time going to work, adopting the new changes I recommend in the plan so that you will get the results you desire and find yourself in a position where you feel like you finally have control not just of your waistline, but those small and large decisions that give life meaning.

Let me be clear—NO ONE is perfect. I've never met the perfect person, but if you have, let me know and please make an introduction. I NEVER expect those who follow my plans to be perfect, so I don't ask for it. Besides, think about how boring life would be if it was perfect. I strongly believe what gives life its texture is succeeding and failing, exploring and experimenting, learning lessons as well as teaching them.

Basically, all that I ask is that you're honest with yourself and do your best. If you decide you only want to follow the plan half the time, please don't expect to get the best results. Be honest. You gave 50% effort so expect less than optimal outcomes. I'm not angry at you or reprimanding you for doing less than your best. For a variety of reasons, sometimes in life we simply don't give our best effort. That's just the way life is sometimes. The key, however, is to match your expectations with your effort.

One more thing before I go—please remember that this plan, like any plan is just a blueprint. It is not a guarantee of what will happen or how much weight you will lose. That part is left to the construction team that builds the structure *based* on the blueprint. You are the construction worker and the plan on these pages is the blueprint. You follow it as best as you can, but there are times you might decide to make some different choices that better suit where you are at the moment or what you want. That's completely fine. I want to give you agency to make those changes so that you wholly own the final structure you build. Sometimes that structure might be a masterpiece and sometimes it might be something quite ordinary. The point is that regardless of what it turns out to be, it's yours. Own it unapologetically, and if you truly don't like it, nothing is stopping you from trying all over again. There's nothing like a great comeback!

GO BUILD THAT TEMPLE!

Ian K. Smith, MD
December 2021

CHAPTER 1

THE GIST: HOW IT WORKS

I have designed this book to be one of the easiest books you'll ever have to read when it comes to weight loss. The basic premise of **BURN MELT SHRED** is one word—**EASY**! I don't want to inundate you with a bunch of extraneous information that you probably already know or don't have a lot of time to read. This book is all about delivering what you need to transform not just your body but also your mind.

The key to this plan is to treat each week separately. Think about each week being a trip to a new foreign place. Keep your excitement and energy high. Be open to new adventures as you explore. Be realistic and accept that every experience is not going to be the best, but enjoy the process and appreciate the opportunity you have to try something different, even if it's not something you want to try again.

I have written the plan in a manner that is straightforward. Each week starts with a set of guidelines. No set of guidelines can ever by complete. There are always scenarios and conditions and exceptions and special circumstances. I can't predict all of these for everyone, so I have done my best to cover the basic ground rules. The rest I'm leaving up to you to make reasonable decisions and use common sense. The way the program works is as it's laid out. Go day by day, week by week and get through the program as best as you can. I've been told by thousands of people over the years, just tell me what to eat, how to eat it, and when to eat it. Take out the guesswork. Well, that's exactly what I've done. To that end, I want to make a few points that will guide you as you **BURN, MELT,** and **SHRED!**

▲I am offering you help outside of this book. I am making myself available on two platforms so you can reach out to me.

BURN MELT SHRED

1. Facebook. I have set up a Facebook group where all of us can congregate and help each other and discuss the plan. I can answer questions and make comments as often as I can. The name of that group is.. you guessed it… **BURN MELT SHRED**. So search for that group on Facebook and click the link requesting to join the group and you will be let in.

2. My Instagram page has a lot of nutrition and fitness information (as well as some great travel videos and photographs—check out the safari stuff, it's awesome) that can help you. You can also send me a DM on Instagram. My handle is @doctoriansmith. Make sure you follow me. Please be patient when sending me messages as I try to get to all of them as fast as possible.

▲ There are some specific exercises listed within the daily meal plan. Obviously, if you need or want to do different exercises, by all means you're free to do that. The most important thing is to pay attention to the suggested time of the exercise. Try to at least fulfill the time suggestion even if you do a different exercise.

▲ A serving of veggies is typically the size of an adult's fist. Will you mess up the plan if you eat a little more. Of course, not. We're talking veggies after all, so it's all good and there aren't many calories involved unless you fry them in oil—something that you're not going to do, right?

▲ Some people have medical conditions, food allergies, food restrictions, food access challenges. I understand that completely. If you have any of these considerations, please make substitutions where necessary. Try to keep your calories under control with the substitutions and you'll be fine.

▲ If you want to remove things from the menu items, that is fine. For example, if you want a burger, but you don't want the bun or you don't want the fish or chicken on top of your salad or the rice with your vegetables—it's always fine to remove items as they are optional.

▲ At the end of the 8 weeks, don't stop. Even if you've hit your goal, still do another 2 weeks and lose a few more pounds to give yourself a cushion. If you still need to lose more weight, please do another 8-week cycle. You might even want to mix up the order of the weeks. That is completely fine. Keep doing various weeks of the diet until you have reached your goal.

▲ No one wants to be on a strict diet forever, so learn how to make better choices as your going through the plan and figure out what works for you and what doesn't. My hope is that you won't constantly need the book to know what to eat, but you will develop the instincts to know what is best to eat and the appropriate portions.

▲ If you mess up a meal or day on the plan, don't stress out. This plan is not at all about stress. Feel free to re-do a day if you feel like it didn't go well, and just keep marching on. This is not a program that penalizes you for mistakes. There's flexibility and forgiveness written into the plan because we're all human and no one is perfect.

▲ There are lots of snacks in the back of the book and some listed on specific days. Try your best to use those snacks, but if for some reason you can't access them, feel free to snack out of the book, but make sure you're keeping the calorie count within the proper range listed in the meal plan. Be a smart snacker. Sure, you can have 2 chocolate chip cookies to meet your 150 calories, but that is not smart snacking as you are getting all sugar and it won't keep you full long. Try snacks that have more protein and fiber as they will keep you full longer.

▲ Everyone who is changing their diet and exercise regimen should definitely talk to their personal doctor and/or other health care provider to make sure this is something you should do and it's safe for you. You might have a condition that puts certain restrictions or considerations on what you can eat or what exercises you can do, so check with your doctor to make sure the plan is alright for you.

▲ Have fun. That's the most important thing. Life is too short, and we face too many difficulties on this journey not to have as much fun as possible!

CHAPTER 2

Week 1

"Bricks become walls and walls become rooms and

rooms become mansions, but regardless of how glorious

the end result, the work started with just one brick."

GUIDELINES

♦If you don't eat meat, make the substitutions appropriately with
fish or vegetables.

♦3 alcoholic drinks allowed per week

♦Soups can be consumed with 2 saltine crackers if desired.

♦The liquid meals must be eaten with either 1 piece of fruit or 1 serving of vegetables.

♦You must consume 1 cup of water before eating a meal; you must consume 1 cup of water during your meal. You can add lemon or lime to your water, and you can drink fizzy water if you desire.

♦You are allowed to drink coffee, but only 2 cups per day. Stay away from those fancy coffee preparations that add a lot of calories. Your coffee should contain no more than 50 calories

♦Don't eat your first meal until 2 hours after you are awake.

♦Do not eat the last meal within 2 hours of going to sleep. You can eat a 100-calorie snack before going to bed if desired.

♦Be smart in your snack choices. Avoid chips, doughnuts, and candy; you can have them some of the time, but don't eat them often. They must fall within the calorie limit as described in the daily meal plan if you decide to have them, but please note these are not smart snacks nor beneficial to your long-term goals. If you must have something like these items, make it only one of your snacks for the day and use healthier options for the other snacks.

♦You don't have to eat all of the food on the day's menu if you don't want to, but no skipping meals, no doubling up on meals, and no exceeding the meal guidelines in size and volume.

♦Condiments such as ketchup, mayo, and mustard are allowed but no more than a teaspoon at each meal. The same goes for soy sauce.

♦You can consume unlimited spices.

♦While fresh fruit is always preferred, canned and frozen fruit are allowed. Just make sure they are water-based and there are no added sugars.

♦Canned and frozen vegetables are allowed. Please be aware of the sodium content.

♦As far as beverages are concerned, you are allowed as much water as you like per day. Here are some other beverage guidelines:

*Flavored waters allowed, but keep them under 60 calories

*1 bottle of sports drink allowed per day, but keep under 60 calories

♦NO WHITE BREAD

♦NO SODA

♦NO FRIED FOOD

♦NO WHITE PASTA (except in the case of chicken noodle soup)

BURN MELT SHRED
DAY 1

Meal 1

Choose one of the following:

•1 small bowl of oatmeal (1.5 cups cooked) with 1 piece of fruit

•2 egg whites or I egg-white omelet with diced veggies (made with

2 egg whites max) with 1 piece of fruit

•1 small bowl of sugar-free cereal with fat-free, skim, or 1-percent

fat milk with 1 piece of fruit

•One 8-ounce yogurt parfait with berries and ⅓ cup granola with 1

piece of fruit

Snack 1: 100 calories or less

Meal 2

Choose one of the following:

•1 large green garden salad with 3 oz of chicken or fish if desired.

(Only 3 tablespoons of fat-free dressing, no bacon bits, no

croutons. Keep it clean.)

•1½ cups of soup (lentil, black bean, white bean, tomato, or cucumber)

•Chicken sandwich on 100% whole-wheat or whole grain bread with lettuce, tomato, 1 slice of cheese, and 1 tbsp of your preferred condiment

Snack 2: 150 calories or less

Meal 3

Choose one of the following:

•One 6-oz piece of grilled or baked chicken or fish with two servings of veggies

•One grilled or baked pork chop and 2 servings of vegetables

•1½ cups whole grain spaghetti with all, some, or none of the following (diced zucchini, squash, peppers, tomatoes, broccoli) in a marina or lemon-wine sauce)

•Portobello mushroom steaks (first marinade in spices and soy sauce or balsamic vinaigrette with a touch of olive oil to cook in and salt and pepper to taste)

Snack 3: 100 calories or less

EXERCISE

•Minimum 30 minutes. If you want to do more, all the better! Work as hard as you can!

Choose a combination of the items below to fulfill your exercise requirement. For those who don't have access to a gym, there are non-gym exercises below.

Gym Exercises

DO TWO OF THE FOLLOWING:

•15 minutes walking/running on treadmill

•15 minutes on elliptical machine

•15 minutes on stationary or mobile bicycle

•15 minutes swimming laps

•15 minutes on stair climber

•20 minutes treadmill intervals

•15 minutes of Zumba

•15 minutes of spinning

•15 minutes of any other high-intensity cardio

•15 minutes of rowing machine

Non-Gym Exercises

DO TWO OF THE FOLLOWING:

•Marching high knees (Stand in position, pump your arms by your side as you alternatively lift your knees up into the air until they just break parallel. Think about soldiers marching in place)—30 seconds continuous knee pumps followed by 40 seconds of rest. This is the equivalent of one set. Do 10 sets in row.

•225 jump rope revolutions

•15 minutes jogging outside

•15 minutes speed walking outside

•Jog punches (Run in place and punch the air above your head with alternating punches) 30 seconds of exercise followed by 40 second of rest. This is the equivalent of one set. Do 10 sets in a row.

DAY 2

Meal 1

•Must have 1 piece of fruit with all of the choices below except the shake. This can be 1 banana, 1 apple, 1 pear, etc. It can also be ½ cup of raspberries, blueberries, blackberries, or straw- berries.

Choose one of the following. Your portion should measure 1 cup after being cooked.

•1 small bowl of oatmeal

•1 small bowl of Cream of Wheat 1 small bowl of grits

•8-oz yogurt parfait

•12-oz protein shake (350 calories or less)

Snack 1: 150 calories or less

Meal 2

Choose one of the following. Your choice must be 300 calories or less.

•1 bowl of soup (no potatoes, no cream) with 1 serving of veggies. Good choices are chicken noodle, vegetable, lentil, chickpea, split pea, black bean, tomato bisque, etc. Be careful of sodium content.

•1 veggie and hummus sandwich on 100% whole-grain or whole-wheat bread

•burrito bowl—1½ cups—brown rice, beans of your choice, tomato, avocado, onion, shredded lettuce

Snack 2: 150 calorie or less

Meal 3

Choose one of the following.

•6-ounce piece of chicken (no skin, no frying) with ½ cup of brown rice and 1 vegetable

•6-ounce piece of fish (no frying) with ½ cup of brown rice and 1 vegetable

•6-ounce piece of turkey (no skin, no frying) with ½ cup of brown rice and 1 vegetable

•One grilled or baked pork chop with ½ cup of brown rice and 1 vegetable

•4 servings of vegetables

Snack 3: 150 calories or less

EXERCISE

•12,000 steps throughout the day. Use your wearable device or smart phone to keep track.

DAY 3

Meal 1

Choose 1 of the following (must be 250 calories or less)

•1 fruit smoothie

•1 veggie smoothie (You can use any veggies you want.)

•1 protein shake

•1 cup steel-cut oats (optional: berries, bananas, cinnamon) with 2 slices of bacon optional with 1 piece of fruit

•1 cup cold cereal with 1 piece of fruit

Snack 1: 150 calorie or less

Meal 2

Choose one of the following:

•3 servings of vegetables (Remember, a serving is about the size of the average person's fist.) One of the vegetables must be a dark-green leafy vegetable, such as spinach, kale, lettuce, mustard greens, collard greens, chicory, or Swiss chard. One must also be some type of legume (lentils, peas, chickpeas, soybeans, black

30

beans, white beans, red beans, lima beans, mung beans, pinto

beans, navy beans, black-eyed peas, etc.)

•1 large green garden salad with ½ cup of legumes (no croutons,

no bacon bits, 3 tablespoons of fat-free or low-fat dressing)

•1 cup of brown rice or quinoa with½ cup of legumes

•1 cup of soup with 1 serving of vegetables. Avoid creamy soups.

Snack 2: 150 calories or less

Meal 3

Choose one of the following.

•1 large green garden salad with 5 oz chicken or fish if desired (no

croutons, no bacon bits, 3 tablespoons of fat-free or low-fat

dressing)

•Serve 6 ounces steamed shrimp or baked fish topped with 3 tbsp

salsa and served with 1 small baked sweet and one serving of green

veggie of your choice

•1 bowl of soup (300 calories or less; no potatoes, no cream) with

2 servings of veggies

Snack 3: 150 calories or less

EXERCISE

Gym Exercises

DO TWO OF THE FOLLOWING:

•15 minutes walking/running on treadmill

•15 minutes on elliptical machine

•15 minutes on stationary or mobile bicycle

•15 minutes swimming laps

•15 minutes on stair climber

•20 minutes treadmill intervals

•15 minutes of Zumba

•15 minutes of spinning

•15 minutes of any other high-intensity cardio

•15 minutes of rowing machine

Non-Gym Exercises

DO TWO OF THE FOLLOWING:

•Marching high knees (Stand in position, pump your arms by your side as you alternatively lift your knees up into the air until they just break parallel. Think about soldiers marching in place)—30 seconds continuous knee pumps followed by 40 seconds rest. This is the equivalent of one set. Do 10 sets in row.

•225 jump rope revolutions

•15 minutes jogging outside

•15 minutes speed walking outside

•Jog punches (Run in place and punch the air above your head with alternating punches) 30 seconds of exercise followed by 40 second of rest. This is the equivalent of one set. Do 10 sets in a row.

DAY 4

Meal 1

Choose one of the following:

•1 small bowl of oatmeal (1½ cups cooked) with 1 piece of fruit

•2 egg whites *or* 1 egg-white omelet with diced veggies (made with 2 egg whites max)

•1 small bowl of sugar-free cereal with fat-free, skim, or I-percent fat milk with 1 piece of fruit

•1 grilled cheese on 100-percent whole-grain or 100-percent whole-wheat bread with 1 piece of fruit

Snack: 150 calories or less

Meal 2

Choose one of the following:

•1 large green salad w/3 tablespoons of vinaigrette dressing (options: 4 olives, 3 oz shredded cheese, 6 cherry tomatoes, ¼ cup nuts, ½ boiled egg; NO bacon, NO croutons, NO ham)

•Chicken salad on a bed of lettuce; toss 3-4 ounces shredded skinless roast chicken breast with ¼ cup sliced red grapes, 1 tbsp halved almonds, 1 tbsp plain, unsweetened Greek yogurt, and 1 tbsp mayonnaise.

•4 servings of vegetables (Remember, a serving is about the size of the average person's fist.)

•Lettuce, cheese, tomato sandwich on 100% whole-grain or whole-wheat toast with your choice of spread

Snack: 150 calories or less

Meal 3

Choose one of the following:

•4 servings of vegetables, raw or cooked

•1 Protein shake (350 calories or less)

•1 cup of whole grain pasta in a meatless tomato sauce with 1 serving of veggies mixed into the pasta

EXERCISE

•Rest Day

DAY 5

Meal 1

Choose one of the following:

•1 cup low-fat or nonfat plain Greek yogurt with ⅓ cup granola or muesli and ¼ cup berries

•1 protein shake (350 calories or less, no added sugars)

•One 12-oz fruit smoothie (350 calories or less)

Snack: 150 calories or less

Meal 2

Choose one of the following:

•1 large green salad w/3 tablespoons of vinaigrette dressing (options: 4 olives, 3 oz shredded cheese, 6 cherry tomatoes, ¼ cup nuts, ½ boiled egg; NO bacon, NO croutons, NO ham)

•1½ cups of soup (options: black bean, white bean, tomato, gazpacho, lentil, chickpeas, vegetable, squash, pea); NO creamy or potato soups

•1 turkey sandwich or 1 chicken sandwich (1 ounce of sliced meat) on 100 percent whole-grain or whole-wheat bread with a teaspoon of mustard or mayo, a slice of tomato, lettuce, and 1 slice of cheese.

Snack: 150 calories or less

Meal 3

Choose one of the following:

•6 ounces fish (grilled or baked, not fried) with 2 serving of vegetables

•4 servings of vegetables, raw or cooked

•1 large green salad w/3 tablespoons of vinaigrette dressing (options: 4 olives, 3 oz shredded cheese, 6 cherry tomatoes, ¼ cup nuts, ½ boiled egg; NO bacon, NO croutons, NO ham)

EXERCISE

Walk 14,000 steps for the day

Day 6

Meal 1

Choose one of the following:

•6 ounces of low fat, plain yogurt; add sliced fresh fruit

•1 egg-white omelet (made with 2 egg whites or ½ cup of Egg Beaters; little butter or cooking spray is allowed

•1 cup of cold cereal or oatmeal with milk and 1 serving of fruit

•1 large fruit plate (½ sliced apple, ½ sliced grapefruit, 3 slices melon)

*Optional: 1 piece of 100 percent whole grain or whole wheat toast

Snack: 150 calories or less

Meal 2

Choose one of the following:

•4 servings of cooked or raw vegetables

•1½ cups of soup (options: black bean, white bean, tomato, gazpacho, lentil, chickpeas, vegetable, squash, pea); NO creamy or potato soups

Snack: 150 calories or less

Meal 3

Choose one of the following:

•4 servings of vegetables, raw or cooked with 1 cup cooked brown or white rice

•One 6-oz piece of grilled or baked chicken or fish with two servings of veggies

•1 large green salad w/3 tablespoons of vinaigrette dressing (options: 4 olives, 3 oz shredded cheese, 6 cherry tomatoes, ¼ cup nuts, ½ boiled egg; NO bacon, NO croutons, NO ham)

EXERCISE

•Rest Day

DAY 7

Meal 1

Choose one of the following:

•2 pancakes the size of a CD with 2 strips of bacon (turkey)

•2 scrambled eggs (diced veggie and 1 tablespoon shredded cheese optional; little butter or cooking spray allowed)

•1 egg white omelet (2 egg whites or ½ cup Egg Beaters; diced veggies optional) 1 cup of oatmeal

•1 cup of cold cereal

Snack: 150 calories or less

Meal 2

•1 large green salad w/3 tablespoons of vinaigrette dressing (options: 4 olives, 3 oz shredded cheese, 6 cherry tomatoes, ¼ cup nuts, ½ boiled egg; NO bacon, NO croutons, NO ham)

•1 bowl of soup (no potatoes, no cream). Good choices are chicken noodle, vegetable, lentil, chickpea, split pea, black bean, tomato bisque, etc. Be careful of sodium content with 1 serving of veggies

•1 veggie and hummus sandwich on 100% whole-grain or whole-wheat bread

•burrito bowl—1½ cups—brown rice, beans of your choice, tomato, avocado, onion, shredded lettuce

Snack: 150 calories or less

Meal 3

Choose one of the following:

•6-ounce piece of chicken (no skin, no frying) with ½ cup of brown rice and 1 vegetable

•6-ounce piece of fish (no frying) with ½ cup of brown rice and 1 vegetable

•6-ounce piece of turkey (no skin, no frying) with ½ cup of brown rice and 1 vegetable

•4 servings of vegetables

EXERCISE

•40 minutes of cardio broken up into 2 sessions

CHAPTER 3

Week 2

"Find a way to unlock your motivation, and you will have found a way to open the door to your success."

GUIDELINES

♦If you don't eat meat, make the substitutions appropriately with fish or vegetables.

♦3 alcoholic drinks allowed per week

♦Soups can be consumed with 2 saltine crackers if desired.

♦The liquid meals must be eaten with either 1 piece of fruit or 1 serving of vegetables.

BURN MELT SHRED

♦You must consume 1 cup of water before eating a meal; you must consume 1 cup of water during your meal. You can add lemon or lime to your water, and you can drink fizzy water if you desire.

♦You are allowed to drink coffee, but only 2 cups per day. Stay away from those fancy coffee preparations that add a lot of calories. Your coffee should contain no more than 50 calories

♦Don't eat your first meal until 2 hours after you are awake.

♦Do not eat the last meal within 2 hours of going to sleep. You can eat a 100-calorie snack before going to bed if desired.

♦Be smart in your snack choices. Avoid chips, doughnuts, and candy; you can have them some of the time, but don't eat them often. They must fall within the calorie limit as described in the daily meal plan if you decide to have them, but please note these are not smart snacks nor beneficial to your long-term goals. If you must have something like these items, make it only one of your snacks for the day and use healthier options for the other snacks.

♦You can choose snacks from the snacks chapter, however, if it indicates that you must eat snacks from a set list for that day, please choose from that list

♦You don't have to eat all of the food on the day's menu if you don't want to, but no skipping meals, no doubling up on meals, and no exceeding the meal guidelines in size and volume.

♦Condiments such as ketchup, mayo, and mustard are allowed, but no more than a teaspoon at each meal. The same goes for soy sauce.

♦You can consume unlimited spices.

♦While fresh fruit is always preferred, canned and frozen fruit are allowed. Just make sure they are water-based and there are no added sugars.

♦Canned and frozen vegetables are allowed. Please be aware of the sodium content.

♦As far as beverages are concerned, you are allowed as much water as you like per day. Here are some other beverage guidelines:

BURN MELT SHRED

♦Flavored waters allowed, but keep them under 60 calories

♦1 bottle of sports drink allowed per day, but keep under 60 calories

♦1-2 beers *or* 1 mixed drink every other day (e.g., on Monday you can have 2 beers, but nothing on Tuesday, then you can have a drink on Wednesday, etc.)

♦NO WHITE BREAD

♦NO SODA

♦NO FRIED FOOD

♦NO WHITE PASTA (except in the case of chicken noodle soup)

DAY 1

Meal 1

Choose one of the following:

• 1 protein shake (350 calories or less, no added sugars)

• 1 12-ounce fruit smoothie (350 calories or less)

• 2 scrambled eggs with cheese and vegetables

Snack: 150 calories or less

Meal 2

• 1 large green salad with 3 tablespoons vinaigrette dressing (options: 4 olives, 3 ounces shredded cheese, 6 cherry tomatoes, 1/4 cup nuts, 1/2 boiled egg; no bacon, no croutons, no ham)

• 1½ cups black bean, white bean, corn, vegetable, tomato, miso, or onion soup

Snack: 150 calories or less

Meal 3

Choose one of the following:

•4 servings of vegetables, raw or cooked with one cup cooked brown or white rice

•1 cup cooked whole-grain pasta in a meatless tomato sauce with 1 serving of veggies mixed into the pasta

•2 cups soup with small green garden salad (soup options: black bean, white bean, tomato, gazpacho, lentil, chickpeas, vegetable, squash, pea, cabbage); no creamy or potato soups

EXERCISE

•30 minutes of cardio/resistance training

DAY 2

Meal 1

Choose one of the following:

•1 protein shake (350 calories or less, no added sugars)

•One 12-ounce fruit smoothie (350 calories or less, no added sugars)

•One 8-ounce yogurt parfait with low-fat plain Greek yogurt, ¼ cup granola or nuts, and ⅓ cup berries

•1 fruit plate (3 servings of fruit)

•1½ cups cold or hot cereal with ½ cup berries or ½ banana sliced

Snack: 150 calories or less

Meal 2

Choose one of the following:

•1 large green salad with 3 tablespoons vinaigrette dressing (options: 4 olives, 3 ounces shredded cheese, 6 cherry tomatoes, ¼ cup nuts, ½ boiled egg; no bacon, no croutons, no ham)

•Chicken or turkey sandwich on 100 percent whole-grain or 100 percent whole-wheat bread with tomato, lettuce, and cheese optional and 2 teaspoons of your preferred condiments

Snack: 150 calories or less

Meal 3

Choose one of the following:

•4 servings of vegetables, raw or cooked

•1 large green salad with 3 tablespoons vinaigrette dressing (options: 4 olives, 3 ounces shredded cheese, 6 cherry tomatoes, 1/4 cup nuts, 1/2 boiled egg; no bacon, no croutons, no ham)

•2 slices pizza with a small green garden salad

EXERCISE

•14,000 steps over the course of the entire day

•5 minutes of running or walking quickly in place, making sure you pump your arms

•20 squats (Do 5 squats consecutively and do that 4 times. If you are unable to do that, sit down and get up from a chair as a modification.)

DAY 3

Meal 1

Choose one of the following:

•1½ cups whole-grain cereal with berries and oat, soy, or almond milk

•1 slice mashed avocado toast on 100 percent whole-grain or 100 percent whole-wheat bread

•1½ cups overnight oats with fresh fruit

•3–4 servings of fruit

Snack: 100 calories or less

Choose one of the following:

•2 frozen fruit bars (no sugar added)

•3 cups air-popped popcorn

•10 black olives

•½ cup quinoa or brown rice

•5 baby carrots and 3 tablespoons hummus

Meal 2

Choose one of the following:

•1 ½ cups creamy tomato soup

•1 ½ cups chicken noodle soup

•Chicken or turkey club sandwich on 100 percent whole-grain or 100 percent whole-wheat bread with lettuce, tomato, onion, and cheese and 2 teaspoons condiment of your choice

Snack: 150 calories or less

Choose one of the following:

•¾ cup roasted chickpeas

•2 cups watermelon chunks

•Apricots and almonds (4 dried apricot halves with 15 dry-roasted almonds)

•½ small apple, sliced, with 2 teaspoons organic peanut butter

•Dehydrated cinnamon apples: Thinly slice 3 medium apples. Sprinkle apples with cinnamon. Spread evenly on parchment paper in a baking dish. Place in an oven on low heat (170 degrees) for approximately 5–6 hours, turning them every hour until browned

and crispy. (Eat one apple worth of slices as a snack and save the

other two for later.)

Meal 3

Choose one of the following:

•Whole-grain bowl (1 cup quinoa or brown rice, greens, veggies,

and balsamic vinaigrette drizzle)

•Hummus and veggies in whole-wheat pita pocket (take whole-

wheat pita and cut in half)

•1½ cups vegetable and chickpea stew with 3⁄4 cup roasted

potatoes

Snack: 100 calories or less

Choose one of the following:

•White bean salad: ½ cup white beans, squeeze of lemon juice, ¼

cup diced tomatoes, 4 cucumber slices

•¾ cup roasted cauliflower with pinch of sea salt

•½ medium avocado sprinkled with a little squeeze of lime juice and sea salt

•3 tablespoons tomato dip (put 1 large tomato, ½ clove minced garlic, 2 tablespoons olive oil, 15 almonds in food processor and blend) and 4 pita wedges

EXERCISE

•Rest Day

Meal 1

Choose one of the following:

•Smoothie (300 calories or less)

•8 ounces soy-based yogurt with granola and strawberries or blueberries (check nutrition label to make sure there isn't a lot of sugar: 5 grams or less)

•1 cup chia seed pudding with banana slices

Snack: 100 calories or less

Choose one of the following:

•16 saltines

•½ cup avocado topped with diced tomatoes and a pinch of pepper

•21 raw almonds

•3/4 cup roasted cauliflower with pinch of sea salt

•10 baby carrots dipped in 2 tablespoons light salad dressing

Meal 2

Choose one of the following:

•6 ounces salmon with 2 servings of vegetables or small salad

•Energy bowl: Combine in a bowl 1/2 cup diced chicken, 1/2 cup brown rice, 1/4 cup cubed cucumber, 1/4 cup halved cherry tomatoes, 2 thin avocado slices, 2 tablespoons balsamic vinaigrette.

•Greek salad topped with 3 ounces sliced fish or chicken

Snack: 150 calories or less

Choose one of the following:

•1 fat-free mozzarella cheese stick with ½ medium apple, sliced (keep skin on)

•1 medium red bell pepper, sliced, with 2 tablespoons soft goat cheese

•½ cup diced cantaloupe topped with ½ cup low-fat cottage cheese

•3 ounces tuna, canned in water

•2 ounces lean roast beef

Meal 3

BURN MELT SHRED

Choose one of the following:

•6-ounce piece of garlic lemon herb chicken with roasted

vegetables and ½ cup potatoes

•1½ cups whole-wheat pasta with diced chicken or fish

•Grilled or baked pork chop with 2 servings of vegetables

Snack: 100 calories or less

Choose one of the following:

•1 cup cherries

•1 piece of fruit of your choice (apple, banana, pear, orange, etc.)

•2 small peaches

•1/3 cup wasabi peas or edamame

•1 large raw carrot

•1 cup mixed berries

EXERCISE

•35 minutes of cardio broken up into 2 sessions (try to do one in

the morning and one in the late afternoon/early evening. A brisk

walk can suffice for the section session)

DAY 5

Meal 1

Choose one of the following:

• 1 protein shake (350 calories or less, no added sugars)

• One 12-ounce fruit smoothie (350 calories or less)

• 1 large fruit plate (½ sliced apple, ½ sliced grapefruit, 3 slices melon)

• 1 bowl cold cereal with 1 cup low-fat milk and a piece of fruit

• One 8-ounce yogurt parfait with low-fat plain Greek yogurt, ¼ cup granola or nuts and 1/3 cup berries

Snack: 150 calories or less

Meal 2

• 1 large green salad with 3 tablespoons vinaigrette dressing (options: 4 olives, 3 ounces shredded cheese, 6 cherry tomatoes, ¼ cup nuts, ½ boiled egg; no bacon, no croutons, no ham)

•1½ cups soup (options: black bean, white bean, tomato, gazpacho, lentil, chickpeas, vegetable, squash, pea, cabbage); no creamy or potato soups

•1 meatless burrito (beans, brown rice, guacamole, shredded cheese) in a whole-grain tortilla

Snack: 150 calories or less

Meal 3

Choose one of the following:

•4 servings of vegetables, raw or cooked, with 1 cup cooked brown rice

•1 protein shake (350 calories or less)

•1 cup whole-grain pasta in a meatless tomato sauce with 1 serving of veggies mixed into the pasta

•One 6-ounce piece of grilled or baked chicken or fish with 2 servings of vegetables

•One grilled or baked pork chop and 2 servings of vegetables

•1 saucy sloppy joe and a serving of vegetables or small green

garden salad (see recipe in RECIPES chapter)

EXERCISE

•30 minutes of cardio/resistance training

DAY 6

Meal 1

Choose one of the following:

•1 protein shake (350 calories or less, no added sugars)

•One 12-ounce fruit smoothie (350 calories or less)

•1 large fruit plate (½ sliced apple, ½ sliced grapefruit, 3 slices melon)

•1 bowl cold or hot cereal with 1 cup low-fat milk and a piece of fruit

Snack: 150 calories or less

Meal 2

•1 large green salad with 3 tablespoons vinaigrette dressing (options: 4 olives, 3 ounces shredded cheese, 6 cherry tomatoes, ¼ cup nuts, ½ boiled egg; no bacon, no croutons, NO ham)

•1½ cups soup (options: black bean, white bean, tomato, gazpacho, lentil, chickpeas, vegetable, squash, pea, cabbage); no creamy or potato soups

•1 protein shake (350 calories or less, no added sugars)

•1 veggie burger on whole-grain bun with lettuce, tomato, cheese optional and 2 teaspoons condiments

Snack: 150 calories or less

Meal 3

Choose one of the following:

•4 servings of vegetables, raw or cooked with 1 cup cooked brown or white rice

•1 protein shake (350 calories or less)

•1 cup whole-grain pasta in a meatless tomato sauce with 1 serving of veggies mixed into the pasta

•6 ounces grilled or baked fish with 2 servings of vegetables

•6 ounces grilled or baked chicken nicely seasoned with 2 servings of vegetables

EXERCISE

•Rest Day

DAY 7

Meal 1

Choose one of the following:

•Avocado toast with sunflower seeds: Spread ½ avocado on 100 percent whole-grain or 100 percent whole-wheat bread, then top with 2 small slices tomato and 1 tablespoon sunflower seeds.

•Raspberry chia parfait: Mash ½ cup raspberries with 1 tablespoon chia seeds, then add to 8 ounces low-fat or fat-free plain yogurt and top with walnuts or pecans.

•2 scrambled eggs with optional cheese and 2 small turkey or pork sausage links or 2 strips turkey or pork bacon. Eat with 1 serving of fruit of your choice.

Snack: 100 calories or less

Choose one of the following:

•3 pineapple rings in natural juices, no sugar added

•10 baby carrots with 2 tablespoons hummus

•White bean salad: ⅓ cup white beans, squeeze of lemon juice, ¾ diced tomatoes, 4 cucumber slices

•1 nectarine

•3–4 tablespoons dried cherries

Meal 2

Choose one of the following:

• Black bean wrap with avocado, diced tomato, lettuce, and brown rice on whole-grain tortilla

• Large green salad (all or any of the following: lettuce, 5 olives, 3 tablespoons shredded cheese, 5 cherry tomatoes, 2 tablespoons nuts, sliced cucumbers) with 2 tablespoons low-fat or fat-free vinaigrette-type dressing

Snack: 150 calories or less

Choose one of the following:

•8–10 slices cucumber and 2 tablespoons hummus

•Watermelon and honeydew melon balls (8 total)

•1 slice 100 percent whole-wheat or whole-grain pita bread, cut up in quarters, with 2 tablespoons hummus

•2 cups air-popped popcorn drizzled with rosemary lemon combo made from combining and heating 2 teaspoons olive oil, 2 teaspoons rosemary, 1/4 teaspoon lemon zest, pinch of sea salt

•Homemade trail mix: Combine 7 roasted almonds, 2 tablespoons dried cranberries, 5 mini pretzel twists, tablespoon shelled sunflower seeds.

Meal 3

Choose one of the following:

•6-ounce piece of grilled or baked fish with 2 servings of vegetables

•6-ounce piece of grilled or baked chicken breast (no skin) with 2 servings of vegetables

•1 piece of layered meat lasagna (4 inches × 3 inches × 2 inches) with small garden salad or 2 servings of vegetables

Snack: 100 calories or less

BURN MELT SHRED

Choose one of the following:

• 16 saltines

• ½ cup avocado topped with diced tomatoes and a pinch of pepper

• 21 raw almonds

• 20 frozen grapes

• Sweet walnut oatmeal (½ cup steel-cut oats cooked with water, topped with 1 tablespoon chopped walnuts and drizzled with teaspoon organic honey or 100 percent maple syrup)

EXERCISE

• 14,000 steps through the course of the day

• 5 minutes of body weight exercises such as jumping jacks/marching in place/stepping up and down from a stair

• 10 minutes of dumbbell curls using light enough weights where you can do 10 repetitions with each arm for 3 sets. Take a 2-minute rest between each set. (If you don't have weights, use bags of flour or rice.)

CHAPTER 4

Week 3

"The body is meant to move just like a sports car is

meant to be driven fast!"

GUIDELINES

♦Drink 1 cup of water before every meal! Do not take your first

bite until you have finished the entire cup.

♦Your first meal can't be eaten before 3 hours after getting up.

Regardless of how many meals you have for that day, your last

meal must be completed BEFORE two hours of going to sleep. So, if you go to sleep at 10 PM, your last meal must be completed by 8 PM.

♦Do your workout before you eat your first meal (fasted workout). Make sure to hydrate before the workout. If you need some energy, you can have an 8 oz yogurt or piece of fruit 30 minutes before the workout

♦2 cups of coffee allowed each day (drink as cleanly as possible— don't load with creams and too much sugar and extra calories; use just a little)

♦Drink one cup of lemon water—hot or cold—each day. You choose the time.

♦If you are a vegan or vegetarian, you can, of course, eliminate the animal products and make substitutions accordingly. However, please try to eat as many high protein non-animal foods as possible when make the substitutions

♦Snacks must come from SNACKS chapter

♦Organic or raw, unfiltered honey is allowed

♦Organic 100% Stevia is allowed

♦NO artificial sweeteners

♦NO Frying—except the stir-fry veggies in olive oil

♦NO white bread

♦NO soda

♦NO white pasta

♦1 serving alcohol allowed each day

BURN MELT SHRED
DAY 1

Meal 1

Choose one of the following:

•1 small bowl of oatmeal (1½ cups cooked) with 1 piece of fruit

•2 egg whites *or* egg-white omelet with diced veggies (made with 2 egg whites max)

•1 small bowl of sugar-free cereal with fat-free, skim, or I-percent fat milk with 1 piece of fruit

•1 grilled cheese on 100-percent whole-grain or 100-percent whole-wheat bread with 1 piece of fruit

Snack: 150 calories or less

Meal 2

•1 large green salad w/3 tablespoons of vinaigrette dressing (options: 4 olives, 3 oz shredded cheese, 6 cherry tomatoes, ¼ cup nuts, ½ boiled egg; NO bacon, NO croutons, NO ham)

•Chicken salad on a bed of lettuce; toss 3-4 ounces shredded skinless roast chicken breast with ¼ cup sliced red grapes, 1 tbsp halved almonds, 1 tbsp plain, unsweetened Greek yogurt, and 1 tbsp mayonnaise.

•4 servings of vegetables (Remember, a serving is about the size of the average person's fist.)

•Lettuce, cheese, tomato sandwich on 100% whole-grain or whole-wheat toast with your choice of spread

Snack: 150 calories or less

Meal 3

Choose one of the following:

•4 servings of vegetables, raw or cooked

•1 Protein shake (350 calories or less)

•1 cup of whole grain pasta in a meatless tomato sauce with 1 serving of veggies mixed into the pasta

EXERCISE

30 minutes of mixed cardio and resistance training

DAY 2

Meal 1

•You must consume 1 piece of fruit with all of the choices below except the shake. This can be 1 banana, 1 apple, 1 pear, etc. It can also be ½ cup of raspberries, blueberries, blackberries, or strawberries.

Choose one of the following. Your portion should be 1 cup cooked.

•1 small bowl of oatmeal

•1 small bowl of Cream of Wheat 1 small bowl of grits

•8-oz yogurt parfait

•12-oz protein shake (350 calories or less)

Snack: 150 calories or less

Meal 2

Choose one of the following. Your choice must be 300 calories or less.

•1 bowl of soup (no potatoes, no cream) with 1 serving of veggies. Good choices are chicken noodle, vegetable, lentil, chickpea, split pea, black bean, tomato bisque, etc. Be careful of sodium content.

•1 veggie and hummus sandwich on 100% whole-grain or whole-wheat bread

•burrito bowl—1½ cups—brown rice, beans of your choice, tomato, avocado, onion, shredded lettuce

Snack 2: 150 calorie or less

Meal 3

•Choose one of the following.

•6-ounce piece of chicken (no skin, no frying) with ½ cup of brown rice and 1 vegetable

•6-ounce piece of fish (no frying) with ½ cup of brown rice and 1 vegetable

•6-ounce piece of turkey (no skin, no frying) with ½ cup of brown rice and 1 vegetable

•4 servings of vegetables

Snack 3: 150 calories or less

EXERCISE

•12,000 steps throughout the day, and/or 30 minutes of cardio +

strength training. Use your wearable device or smart phone to keep

track.

DAY 3 (Plant-based)

You will be eating four smaller meals today rather than the typical three meals and three snacks. Instead of three snacks, you will have two snacks that you can eat whenever you want throughout the day as long as you eat them within your feeding window.

Meal 1

Choose one of the following:

•One 12-oz fruit smoothie (300 calories or less)

•One 12-oz protein shake (300 calories or less)

•One 8-oz yogurt parfait (300 calories or less)

Meal 2

Choose one of the following:

•1½ cups of soup (no potato or heavy cream soup like clam chowder)

•4 servings of veggies (cooked or raw)

•1 large green salad (optional: olives, 2 tbsp shredded cheese, 5 cherry tomatoes, 2 tbsp of nuts) with 2 tbsp of vinaigrette-type dressing

Meal 3

Choose one of the following:

•1½ cups whole-wheat or whole-grain pasta in a marinara sauce with vegetables (squash, broccoli, tomatoes, etc.)

•1 large green salad with veggies, but no croutons or bacon bits (NO creamy salad dressing)

Meal 4

Choose one of the following:

•1½ cups of soup

•1½ cups whole-wheat or whole-grain pasta in a marinara sauce with vegetables (squash, broccoli, tomatoes, etc.)

•2 small slices of cheese pizza no more than 4 inches at the crust and 5 inches long

2 SNACKS TODAY: 100 calories or less

EXERCISE

•Rest Day

Meal 1

Choose one of the following:

•1 cup plain, low-fat Greek yogurt with fresh fruit

•12 ounces of fresh fruit smoothie (300 calories or less)

•2 egg whites or 1 egg-white omelet with diced veggies (made with 2 egg whites max)

•1 small bowl of sugar-free cereal with fat-free, skim, or 1-percent fat milk ½ cup of fresh juice not from concentrate (grapefruit, apple, orange juice, tomato, carrot, etc.)

Snack: 100 calories or less

Meal 2

Choose one of the following:

•burrito bowl—1½ cups—brown rice, beans of your choice, tomato, avocado, onion, shredded lettuce

•egg salad spread over 1 slice of toasted or untoasted 100% whole-grain or whole-wheat bread (for the egg salad, use eggs, low-fat mayo, dill, mustard, chives, salt and pepper)

Snack: 100 calories or less

Meal 3

Choose one of the following:

•1½ cups of soup (lentil, black bean, white bean, tomato, squash, vegetable, or cucumber)

•2 small roasted vegetable and black bean tacos (5-inch diameter)

Snack: 100 calories or less

EXERCISE

•30 minutes

BURN MELT SHRED
DAY 5 (Plant based)

You will be eating four smaller meals today rather than the typical three meals and three snacks. Instead of three snacks, you will have two snacks that you can eat whenever you want throughout the day as long as you eat them within your feeding window.

Meal 1

Choose one of the following:

•One 12-oz fruit smoothie (300 calories or less)

•One 12-oz protein shake for breakfast (300 calories or less)

Meal 2

Choose one of the following:

•1½ cups of soup (NO creamy soup)

•4 servings of veggies (cooked or raw)

•black bean bowl with brown rice avocado and cheese (1 cup cooked brown rice, ½ cup black beans, ½ small avocado, sliced, and 2 tbsp shredded cheese melted or unmelted)

81

Meal 3

Choose one of the following:

•1 large green salad with veggies, but no croutons or bacon bits (NO creamy salad dressing)

•1 veggie burger on whole grain bun with a slice of cheese and tomato

•Brussels sprouts and brown rice

Meal 4

Choose one of the following:

•1½ cups of soup (No creamy soup)

•3 servings of vegetables (cooked or raw) and 1 cup of brown rice

•1 cup of cooked whole-wheat pasta with your choice of 2-3 veggies and a marinara or lemon white wine sauce

2 SNACKS TODAY: 150 calories or less

EXERCISE

•14,000 steps throughout the day

BURN MELT SHRED
DAY 6

Meal 1

Choose 1 of the following (must be 250 calories or less)

•1 fruit smoothie

•1 veggie smoothie (You can use any veggies you want.)

•1 protein shake

•1 cup steel-cut oats (optional: berries, bananas, cinnamon) with 2 slices of bacon optional with 1 piece of fruit

•1 cup cold cereal with 1 piece of fruit

Snack 1: 150 calorie or less

Meal 2

Choose one of the following:

•3 servings of vegetables (Remember, a serving is about the size of the average person's fist.) One of the vegetables must be a dark-green leafy vegetable, such as spinach, kale, lettuce, mustard greens, collard greens, chicory, or Swiss chard. One must also be some type of legume (lentils, peas, chickpeas, soybeans, black beans, white beans, red beans, lima beans, mung beans, pinto

beans, navy beans, black-eyed peas, etc.)

•1 large green garden salad with ½ cup of legumes (no croutons,

no bacon bits, 3 tablespoons of fat-free or low-fat dressing)

•1 cup of brown rice or quinoa with ½ cup of legumes

•1 cup of soup with 1 serving of vegetables. Avoid creamy soups.

Snack 2: 150 calories or less

Meal 3

Choose one of the following.

•1 large green garden salad with 5 oz chicken or fish if desired (no

croutons, no bacon bits, 3 tablespoons of fat-free or low-fat

dressing)

•Serve 6 ounces steamed shrimp or baked fish topped with 3 tbsp

salsa and served with 1 small baked sweet and one serving of green

veggie of your choice

•1 bowl of soup (300 calories or less; no potatoes, no cream) with

2 servings of veggies

Snack 3: 150 calories or less

EXERCISE

•Rest Day

DAY 7 (Plant-based)

You will be eating four smaller meals today rather than the typical three meals and three snacks. Instead of three snacks, you will have two snacks that you can eat whenever you want throughout the day as long as you eat them within your feeding window.

Meal 1

Choose one of the following:

•One 12-oz fruit smoothie (300 calories or less)

•One 12-oz protein shake (300 calories or less)

•One 8-oz yogurt parfait (300 calories or less)

Meal 2

Choose one of the following:

•1½ cups of soup (no potato or heavy cream soup like clam chowder)

•4 servings of veggies (cooked or raw)

•1 large green salad (optional: olives, 2 tbsp shredded cheese, 5 cherry tomatoes, 2 tbsp of nuts) with 2 tbsp of vinaigrette-type dressing

Meal 3

Choose one of the following:

•1½ cups whole-wheat or whole-grain pasta in a marinara sauce with vegetables (squash, broccoli, tomatoes, etc.)

•1 large green salad with veggies, but no croutons or bacon bits (NO creamy salad dressing)

Meal 4

Choose one of the following:

•1½ cups of soup

•1½ cups whole-wheat or whole-grain pasta in a marinara sauce with vegetables (squash, broccoli, tomatoes, etc.)

•2 small slices of cheese pizza no more than 4 inches at the crust and 5 inches long

2 SNACKS TODAY: 100 calories or less

EXERCISE

•Rest Day

CHAPTER 5

Week 4

"Anything worth having in life is worth fighting for."

GUIDELINES

◆No soda or alcohol this week.

◆You can choose snacks from the chapter in the back of the book, however, if a particular day says that you must choose a snack from the list written for that day, please follow those directions

◆You must drink a cup of water before taking the first bite of each meal.

♦You must exercise 4 times this week doing 30 mins at least of exercise each session (You can also break it up into 2 fifteen-minute sessions)

♦You must choose a consecutive 10-hour window where you will eat all of your meals. The other fourteen ours will be your fasting window and you can only drink beverages as long as the total calorie count for all the beverages you drink doesn't surpass 50 calories for that entire fasting window.

♦Work hard and have fun!!

Meal 1

Choose one of the following:

•2 pancakes (5 inches in diameter) with 2 slices turkey or pork bacon

•2 scrambled eggs with optional cheese and 2 small sausage links or 2 strips of turkey or pork bacon. Eat with 1 serving of fruit of your choice.

•2 slices French toast made on 100 percent whole-grain or 100 percent whole-wheat bread and ½ cup berries.

Snack: 150 calories or less

Choose one of the following or a plant-based snacks:

•Applesauce and cereal: 1 applesauce pouch (⅓ cup) and ½ cup dry cereal

•1 medium red bell pepper, sliced, with ¼ cup guacamole

•½ avocado topped with diced tomatoes and a pinch of pepper

•¾ cup roasted black beans

•Small green garden salad (greens, tomatoes, olives, shredded carrots)

Meal 2

Choose one of the following:

•1½ cups tomato, pea, mushroom, or lentil soup and ¾ cup cooked brown rice

•Large green salad (all or any of the following: ½ cup beans, 3 cups lettuce or other greens, 5 olives, 3 tablespoons shredded cheese, 5 cherry tomatoes, 2 tablespoons nuts, sliced cucumbers) with 2 tablespoons low-fat or fat-free vinaigrette-type dressing

Snack 2

Choose one of the following:

•1 slice Swiss cheese and 8 olives

•½ cup light natural vanilla ice cream or sorbet

•1 can water-packed tuna, drained and seasoned to taste

•10 cooked mussels

•½ cup canned crab

Meal 3

Choose one of the following:

•Chicken stir-fry: Cook 6-ounce chicken breast, dice, then set aside. Add ¼ cup diced red bell peppers, ¼ cup diced tomatoes, 1 tablespoon diced onion, 1 clove garlic, minced, and pinch of salt and pepper to skillet. Cook vegetables for approximately 5 minutes while stirring frequently. Add back the chicken and cook for another couple of minutes, then serve.

•Large green salad (all or any of the following: ½ cup beans, 3 cups lettuce or other greens, 5 olives, 3 tablespoons shredded cheese, 5 cherry tomatoes, 2 tablespoons nuts, sliced cucumbers) with 2 tablespoons low-fat or fat-free vinaigrette-type dressing, topped with 3 ounces fish or chicken

•3 giant crab legs with butter sauce dip and 2 servings of vegetables

Snack 3

Choose one of the following:

•Applesauce and cereal: 1 applesauce pouch (⅓ cup) and ½ cup

dry cereal

•10 walnut halves and 1 sliced kiwi

•Baby burrito: 6-inch corn tortilla, 2 tablespoons bean dip, and 2

tablespoons salsa

•1 cup grapes with 10 almonds

•Brown rice vegetable sushi rolls, 5 pieces

Meal 1

Choose one of the following:

•Open-faced egg sandwich: On a whole-grain English muffin or slice of bread, place ⅓ cup cooked sautéed spinach over 1 cooked egg, 1 tablespoon shredded cheese, with salt or pepper to taste. Eat with 1 serving of fruit of your choice.

• 2 whole-wheat pancakes (5 inches in diameter), 2 slices turkey or pork bacon, 1 serving of fruit

• Protein shake (300 calories or less)

Snack 1

Choose one of the following:

•Small baked potato topped with salsa

•¾ cup roasted cauliflower with a pinch of sea salt

•1 cup blueberries with a squirt of whipped cream

•Applesauce and cereal: 1 applesauce pouch (⅓ cup) and ½ cup dry cereal

• 1 medium red bell pepper, sliced, with ¼ cup guacamole

Meal 2

Choose one of the following:

•1½ cups black bean soup, white bean soup, or vegan chili with ¾ cup brown rice

• Large green salad (all or any of the following: ½ cup beans, 3 cups lettuce or other greens, 5 olives, 3 tablespoons shredded cheese, 5 cherry tomatoes, 2 tablespoons nuts, sliced cucumbers) with 2 tablespoons low-fat or fat-free vinaigrette-type dressing

Snack 2

Choose one of the following:

•½ cup pudding of your choice

•3 celery sticks stuffed with cottage cheese (each stick should be 5 inches long)

•1 portobello mushroom stuffed with roasted veggies and 1 teaspoon shredded low-fat cheese

•8 small shrimp and 2 tablespoons cocktail sauce

•1 cup chicken noodle soup

Meal 3

Choose one of the following:

•2 spicy peanut lettuce wraps filled with baked tofu, carrots, cucumbers, peppers, and roasted cauliflower

•1 black bean enchilada and a small garden salad

Snack 3

Choose one of the following:

•½ cup dried apricots

•1½ cups puffed rice

•Watermelon salad: 1 cup raw spinach with ⅔ cup diced watermelon, sprinkled with 1 tablespoon balsamic vinegar

•25 frozen red seedless grapes

DAY 3

Meal 1

Choose one of the following:

• 1½ cups cooked oatmeal or grits with berries or banana

• 2 scrambled eggs (cheese and vegetables optional) and 1 piece of fruit

• Bacon grilled cheese sandwich: Butter one side of 2 pieces of 100 percent whole-grain or 100 percent wholewheat bread, then set aside. Cook 3 slices turkey or pork bacon. Place 1 piece of bread, buttered side down, on a skillet being warmed over medium heat. Place a piece of cheese on top of the bread, then cut the bacon strips in half and place on top of the cheese. Place a second piece of cheese on top of the bacon, then put the second piece of bread on top to complete the sandwich. Make sure the buttered side is facing up. Cook until golden brown and cheese is melting, then flip and cook the second side. Eat warm.

Snack 1

Choose one of the following:

•50 Goldfish crackers

•½ cup kale chips

•⅓ cup low-fat granola

•3 cups air-popped popcorn

•3 tablespoons roasted pumpkin seeds

Meal 2

Choose one of the following:

•1½ cups chicken and rice soup with small green garden salad

•Avocado bacon salad: Chop half a head of romaine lettuce or use 2 cups kale, and place in a bowl. Add ½ cup chopped cucumbers, ¼ cup chopped onions, ½ avocado, sliced. Add 2 slices pork or turkey bacon, diced, then drizzle with 2 tablespoons of your choice of dressing.

•Cucumber tuna salad: Drain 1 can of tuna, then add to a bowl and mix in ½ cup diced cucumbers, skin removed, ½ tablespoon fresh lemon juice, 1 tablespoon mayonnaise, pinch of salt. Serve on a bed of greens or inside a whole-wheat tortilla.

Snack 2

Choose one of the following:

•40 shelled or unshelled pistachios

•¾ cup melon cubes

•1 slice 100 percent whole-grain or whole-wheat pita bread, cut up into quarters, with 2 tablespoons hummus

•1 large apple, orange, or banana

•10 baby carrots

Meal 3

Choose one of the following:

•6 ounces steamed scallops and 2 servings of vegetables

•Chicken stir-fry: Cook 6-ounce chicken breast, dice, then set aside. Add ¼ cup diced red bell peppers, ¼ cup diced tomatoes, 1 tablespoon diced onion, 1 clove garlic, minced, and pinch of salt and pepper to skillet.

•Cook vegetables for approximately 5 minutes while stirring frequently. Add back the chicken and cook for another couple of minutes, then serve.

•2 cups soup of your choice

Snack 3

Choose one of the following:

•¾ cup roasted chickpeas

•¾ cup roasted black beans

•3 hummus-and-veggie roll-ups

•4 almond butter–stuffed dates

•2 tablespoons refried bean dip (made without lard) and 5 tortilla chips

DAY 4

Meal 1

Choose one of the following:

•2 slices French toast made on 100 percent whole-grain or 100 percent whole-wheat bread and ½ cup berries

•8 ounces yogurt topped with berries and ¼ cup granola

•Omelet made with 2 eggs, cheese, and vegetables

Snack 1

Choose one of the following:

•5 pitted dates stuffed with 5 whole almonds

•½ cup unsweetened applesauce mixed with 10 pecan halves

•¼ cup low-fat granola

•1 cup lettuce, drizzled with 2 tablespoons fat-free dressing

•3 oven-baked potato wedges

Meal 2

Choose one of the following:

•Chicken caprese salad: In a large bowl, toss 2 cups greens of your choice, ¾ cup diced chicken, ½ cup mozzarella (or cheese of your choice), ½ cup diced tomato, ¼ cup

chopped fresh basil, 1 teaspoon extra-virgin olive oil, 2

tablespoons fresh lemon juice.

•Power salmon bowl: In a bowl, place 2 cups chopped greens of

your choice, 3 ounces of cooked salmon, chopped, ½ cup diced

cucumbers, ¼ cup shredded carrots, ½ cup diced tomatoes, ½ cup

cooked brown rice. Drizzle with balsamic vinaigrette.

•Turkey or chicken club sandwich on 100 percent whole-grain or

100 percent whole-wheat bread with lettuce, tomato, cheese, and 2

teaspoons of preferred condiments.

Snack 2

Choose one of the following:

•2 frozen fruit bars (no sugar added)

•2 tablespoons hummus spread on 4 crackers

•10 black olives

•½ cup quinoa or brown rice

•5 baby carrots and 3 tablespoons hummus

Meal 3

Choose one of the following:

•3 giant crab legs with butter sauce dip and 2 serving of vegetables

•1 piece of meat lasagna (4 inch × 3 inch × 2 inch) with 2 servings of vegetables

•2 cups chicken or beef stir-fry

Snack 3

Choose one of the following:

•2 cups grilled or roasted broccoli florets

•17 pecans

•25 cherries

•6 dried apricots

•1 rice cake with 1 tablespoon guacamole

BURN MELT SHRED
DAY 5

Meal 1

Choose one of the following:

•2 banana or blueberry pancakes (5-inch diameter) and a serving of breakfast meat (ham or bacon)

•2 scrambled eggs with 3 tablespoons shredded cheese

•1½ cups cold or hot cereal with berries and reduced-fat milk

Snack 1

Choose one of the following:

•½ cup roasted chickpeas

•Small baked potato topped with salsa

•3 cups air-popped popcorn

•½ cup dried apricots

•1½ cups puffed rice

Meal 2

Choose one of the following:

•Large salad with 3 ounces chicken or fish sliced on top

•2 meat tacos with 1 serving of vegetables or small green garden salad

•1½ cups chicken noodle soup with ¾ cup brown rice

Snack 2

Choose one of the following:

•¾ cup roasted chickpeas

•¾ cup roasted black beans

•3 hummus-and-veggie roll-ups

•Apricots and almonds (4 dried apricot halves with 15 dry-roasted almonds)

•½ cup nut-free trail mix with no added sugar

Meal 3

Choose one of the following:

•2 cups vegetarian paella

•4 servings of variety of roasted vegetables with a cup cooked of brown or white rice

Snack 3

Choose one of the following:

•2 tablespoons hummus with 5 baby carrot sticks

•2 tablespoons hummus with ½ small cucumber, sliced

•1 whole-grain waffle topped with 2 tablespoons low-fat or fat-free plain yogurt and ½ cup berries

•Hot quesadilla: Spray one side of corn tortilla with cook spray, then place on a skillet. Top with ¼ cup Mexican cheese blend, fold in half, and cook for a couple of minutes on each side until cheese melts and tortilla has slight crisp. Optional to serve with 2 tablespoons Pico de Gallo or salsa.

•Apple and cottage cheese (small apple, sliced and dipped into ½ cup low-fat cottage cheese and sprinkled with cinnamon)

DAY 6

Meal 1

Choose one of the following:

•Open-faced egg sandwich: On a whole-grain English muffin or slice of bread, place ⅓ cup cooked sautéed spinach over 1 cooked egg, 1 tablespoon shredded cheese, with salt or pepper to taste. Eat with 1 serving of fruit of your choice.

• 2 whole-wheat pancakes (5 inches in diameter), 2 slices turkey or pork bacon, 1 serving of fruit

• Protein shake (300 calories or less)

Snack 1

Choose one of the following:

•Small baked potato topped with salsa

•¾ cup roasted cauliflower with a pinch of sea salt

•1 cup blueberries with a squirt of whipped cream

•Applesauce and cereal: 1 applesauce pouch (⅓ cup) and ½ cup dry cereal

• 1 medium red bell pepper, sliced, with ¼ cup guacamole

Meal 2

Choose one of the following:

•1½ cups black bean soup, white bean soup, or vegan chili with ¾ cup brown rice

• Large green salad (all or any of the following: ½ cup beans, 3 cups lettuce or other greens, 5 olives, 3 tablespoons shredded cheese, 5 cherry tomatoes, 2 tablespoons nuts, sliced cucumbers) with 2 tablespoons low-fat or fat-free vinaigrette-type dressing

Snack 2

Choose one of the following:

•½ cup pudding of your choice

•3 celery sticks stuffed with cottage cheese (each stick should be 5 inches long)

•1 portobello mushroom stuffed with roasted veggies and 1 teaspoon shredded low-fat cheese

•8 small shrimp and 2 tablespoons cocktail sauce

•1 cup chicken noodle soup

Meal 3

Choose one of the following:

•2 spicy peanut lettuce wraps filled with baked tofu, carrots, cucumbers, peppers, and roasted cauliflower

•1 black bean enchilada and a small garden salad

Snack 3

Choose one of the following:

•½ cup dried apricots

•1½ cups puffed rice

•Watermelon salad: 1 cup raw spinach with ⅔ cup diced watermelon, sprinkled with 1 tablespoon balsamic vinegar

•25 frozen red seedless grapes

Meal 1

Choose one of the following:

•2 banana or blueberry pancakes (5-inch diameter) and a serving of breakfast meat (ham or bacon)

•2 scrambled eggs with 3 tablespoons shredded cheese

•1½ cups cold or hot cereal with berries and reduced-fat milk

Snack 1

Choose one of the following:

•½ cup roasted chickpeas

•Small baked potato topped with salsa

•3 cups air-popped popcorn

•½ cup dried apricots

•1½ cups puffed rice

Meal 2

Choose one of the following:

•Large salad with 3 ounces chicken or fish sliced on top

•2 meat tacos with 1 serving of vegetables or small green garden salad

•1½ cups chicken noodle soup with ¾ cup brown rice

Snack 2

Choose one of the following:

•¾ cup roasted chickpeas

•¾ cup roasted black beans

•3 hummus-and-veggie roll-ups

•Apricots and almonds (4 dried apricot halves with 15 dry-roasted almonds)

•½ cup nut-free trail mix with no added sugar

Meal 3

Choose one of the following:

•2 cups vegetarian paella

•4 servings of variety of roasted vegetables with a cup cooked of brown or white rice

Snack 3

Choose one of the following:

•2 tablespoons hummus with 5 baby carrot sticks

•2 tablespoons hummus with ½ small cucumber, sliced

•1 whole-grain waffle topped with 2 tablespoons low-fat or fat-free plain yogurt and ½ cup berries

•Hot quesadilla: Spray one side of corn tortilla with cook spray, then place on a skillet. Top with ¼ cup Mexican cheese blend, fold in half, and cook for a couple of minutes on each side until cheese melts and tortilla has slight crisp. Optional to serve with 2 tablespoons Pico de Gallo or salsa.

•Apple and cottage cheese (small apple, sliced and dipped into ½ cup low-fat cottage cheese and sprinkled with cinnamon)

CHAPTER 6

Week 5

"The body doesn't grow when you think about it, rather

it grows when challenged."

GUIDELINES

♦Drink 1 cup of water before every meal! Do not take your first

bite until you have finished the entire cup.

♦Your first meal can't be eaten before 3 hours after getting up.

Your last meal must be completed BEFORE two hours of going to

sleep. So, if you go to sleep at 10 PM, your last meal must be

completed by 8 PM.

BURN MELT SHRED

◆Do your workout before you eat your first meal (fasted workout). Make sure to hydrate before the workout. If you need some energy, you can have an 8 oz yogurt or piece of fruit 30 minutes before the workout

◆2 cups of coffee allowed each day (drink as cleanly as possible—don't load with creams and too much sugar and extra calories; use just a little)

◆Drink one cup of lemon water—hot or cold—each day. You choose the time.

◆If you are a vegan or vegetarian, you can, of course, eliminate the animal products and make substitutions accordingly. However, please try to eat as many high protein non-animal foods as possible when make the substitutions

◆For your second meal this week, make sure you eat and finish 2 hours before going to sleep.

◆Snacks must come from SNACKS chapter.

◆Organic or raw, unfiltered honey is allowed.

◆Organic 100% Stevia is allowed.

♦NO artificial sweeteners

♦NO Frying—except the stir-fry veggies in olive oil

♦NO white bread

♦NO soda

♦NO white pasta

♦1 serving alcohol allowed each day

DAY 1

*Note: Don't forget that each day you must drink 1 full cup (8 oz) of water before each meal

Meal 1

Choose one of the following:

•1 protein shake (350 calories or less, no sugar added, must contain 10 grams of protein)

•1 fruit smoothie (350 calories or less, no sugar added)

•One 8-oz yogurt parfait with granola and fresh fruit

•1 fruit platter (3 servings of fruit)

Snack: 100 calories or less *Eng muffin half w/t jam*

Snack: 100 calories or less *Baked Potato*

Snack: 150 calories or less *½C Cottage cheese 1 T PB*

Meal 2

Choose one of the following:

•large green garden (optional: tomatoes, peppers, 1 hard-boiled egg, ¼ cup chunked avocado) with 3 tbsp balsamic vinaigrette (add 3 oz of chicken or fish if desired)

•1½ cups of soup (lentil, black bean, white bean, tomato, or

cucumber) with 1 cup of white or brown rice.

4 servings of different vegetables (2 of them must be a legume)

EXERCISE

•30 minutes of combined cardio/resistance training

Meal 1

Choose one of the following:

•2 scrambled eggs with diced veggies, 3 oz cheese and 1 piece of fruit

•1 cup steel-cut oats (optional: berries, bananas, cinnamon) ⟵

Snack: 100 calories or less   ½ C Cottage cheese

Snack: 100 calories or less   3 oz Tuna

Snack: 150 calories or less   2 Egg Salad, ½ Muffin

Meal 2

Choose one of the following:

•1½ cups whole grain spaghetti with all, some, or none of the following (diced zucchini, squash, peppers, tomatoes, broccoli) in a marina or lemon-wine sauce)

•1 serving of 4 different vegetables

EXERCISE

•30 minutes of cardio

Meal 1

Choose one of the following:

•1 protein shake (350 calories or less, no sugar added, must contain 10 grams of protein)

•1 fruit smoothie (350 calories or less, no sugar added)

•One 8-oz yogurt parfait with granola and fresh fruit

•1½ cups of soup

•1 serving of 4 different vegetables (2 must be legumes)

•large green garden with 3 oz of chicken or fish (optional: tomatoes, peppers, 1 hard-boiled egg, ¼ cup chunked avocado) with 3 tbsp balsamic vinaigrette

Snack: 100 calories or less

Snack: 100 calories or less

Snack: 150 calories or less

Meal 2

Choose one of the following:

•1½ cups of vegan or meat chili including onion, red bell pepper, garlic, butternut squash, black beans, pinto beans, and diced tomatoes.

•5 oz turkey burger on whole wheat or whole grain bun with 1 cup baked sweet potato fries or 1 small baked sweet potato

•Large green salad with 3 oz of grilled chicken or seafood

•1½ cups of soup with small green garden salad

•2 cups cooked whole wheat or whole grain pasta with ½ cup diced chicken or fish

EXERCISE

•Rest Day

Meal 1

Choose one of the following:

• 2 slices of avocado toast on 100% whole-wheat or whole-grain bread with 1 serving of fruit

• 1 protein shake (350 calories or less, no sugar added, must contain 10 grams of protein)

• Spinach, onion, and cheese (your choice) scramble on whole-wheat English muffin

• 1 fruit smoothie (350 calories or less, no sugar added)

• One 8-oz yogurt parfait with granola and fresh fruit

Snack: 100 calories or less

Snack: 100 calories or less

Snack: 150 calories or less

Meal 2

Choose one of the following:

• 1½ cups of soup

• 1 serving of 4 different vegetables

•large green garden (optional: tomatoes, peppers, 1 hard-boiled egg, ¼ cup chunked avocado) with 3 tbsp balsamic vinaigrette

•1 medium grilled lamb chop (fat trimmed) with 1 cup mashed cauliflower and 1 cup carrots (or veggie of your choice)

EXERCISE

•30 minutes of combined cardio/resistance training

Meal 1

Choose one of the following:

• 12 oz fresh smoothie (300 calories or less)

• 1 protein shake (350 calories or less, no sugar added; make sure it has 10 grams of protein)

• 1 cup of steel oats with sliced apples and walnuts optional

• Peanut butter and banana sandwich on 100% whole-wheat or whole-grain bread (2 slices whole-wheat bread (2 tbsp organic peanut butter, ½ medium banana sliced, 1 tsp drizzle of raw, unfiltered honey)

• 2 scrambled eggs with cheese, diced veggies and herbs and 2 strips of bacon (turkey or pork)

Snack: 100 calories or less

Snack: 100 calories or less

Snack: 150 calories or less

Meal 2

Choose one of the following:

•3 cups of tomato, cucumber, onion, black or white bean salad with 3 tbsp balsamic vinaigrette with a cup of soup

•Lettuce, cheese, tomato, bacon sandwich on 100% whole-grain or whole-wheat toast with your choice of spread (You can use chicken or ham instead of the bacon) with a cup of soup

•Cauliflower, ground meat and brown rice stuffed peppers (both halves of a small pepper)

•6 oz steak with 2 servings of leafy vegetables

•6 oz grilled or baked chicken or fish with 2 servings of leafy vegetables

•Portobello mushroom steaks (first marinade in spices and soy sauce or balsamic vinaigrette with a touch of olive oil to cook in and salt and pepper to taste) with 2 servings of leafy vegetables

EXERCISE

•30 minutes of combined cardio/resistance training

DAY 6

Meal 1

Choose one of the following:

•2-egg omelet with diced veggies and 3 oz cheese

•12 oz fresh fruit smoothie or protein shake (350 calories or less and shake must contain at least 10 grams of protein)

•Waffle Monte Cristo (spread strawberry or apricot preserves over 2 waffles, layer with turkey, ham, bacon, and cheese, lightly butter outside of waffles, make waffles into sandwich and place on grill on medium heat, 5 minutes each side)

Snack: 100 calories or less

Snack: 100 calories or less

Snack: 150 calories or less

Meal 2

Choose one of the following:

•Bean, vegetable, cheese enchilada on whole-grain tortilla

•6 oz chicken (without skin and not fried)

Small baked sweet potato or dice it to make a cup

1 cup cooked broccoli florets (substitute any green leafy vegetable

•1½ cups Poke bowl with chicken or fish, brown rice, avocado, edamame, cucumber

EXERCISE

•Rest Day

DAY 7

Meal 1

Choose one of the following:

•1 bacon-cheddar grilled cheese sandwich on 100% whole-grain or whole-wheat bread with 1 serving of fruit (You can use different cheese if desired and your choice of bacon or you can eliminate the bacon)

•2-egg omelet with diced veggies and 3 oz cheese

•1 protein shake (350 calories or less, no sugar added, must contain 10 grams of protein)

•1 whole-grain or whole-wheat waffle (8-10 inches diameter) with 2 strips of bacon (turkey or pork) and one serving of fruit

•1½ cups lentil soup (substitute black bean, chickpea, white bean, chicken noodle) with medium green garden salad (2 cups of greens, ½ small cucumber, sliced, ½ small avocado peeled and sliced with diced, ½ cup diced low-fat cheese, 5 cherry tomatoes, halved or whole)

Snack: 100 calories or less

Snack: 100 calories or less

Snack: 150 calories or less

Meal 2

Choose one of the following:

•6 oz salmon (sea bass, cod, branzino, tuna optional) with 1 serving of asparagus (or any leafy green of your choice) and 1 cup cooked brown or white rice

•bean burrito with cheese and sour cream in whole grain flour tortilla (use black or refried beans, low sodium) with 2 servings of vegetables of medium salad

•vegetable stir-fry in olive oil with broccoli, brown rice, peppers, carrots, soy sauce, mushrooms honey (you can add 3 oz of meat if you desire)

EXERCISE

•30 minutes of combined cardio/resistance training

CHAPTER 7

Week 6

"The mind often gives out before the body, so keep your

mental on point and you will stay in the game."

GUIDELINES

♦Drink 1 cup of water before every meal! Do not take your first

bite until you have finished the entire cup.

♦Don't eat your first meal or any solid food until 3 hours after

getting up. Your last meal must be completed BEFORE two hours

of going to sleep

♦For snacks, use the list in the SNACKS chapter.

♦2 cups of coffee allowed each day (drink as cleanly as possible—don't load with creams and too much sugar and extra calories; use just a little)

♦Drink one cup of lemon water—hot or cold—each day. You choose the time.

♦Organic honey allowed

♦Organic 100% Stevia allowed

♦NO artificial sweeteners.

♦NO Frying—except the stir-fry veggies in olive oil

♦NO white bread

♦NO soda

♦NO white pasta

♦1 serving alcohol allowed each day

DAY 1

Meal 1

Choose one of the following:

•2 scrambled eggs with diced veggies, 3 oz cheese and 1 piece of fruit

•1 cup steel-cut oats (optional: berries, bananas, cinnamon)

Snack: 100 calories or less

Meal 2

Choose one of the following:

•large green garden (optional: tomatoes, peppers, 1 hard-boiled egg, ¼ cup chunked avocado) with 3 tbsp balsamic vinaigrette and 3 oz of chicken or fish; if you choose the vegetarian/vegan route and don't want the chick or fish, please make sure you have a cup of beans in your salad

•1½ cups of soup or chili (for the soup, eat lentil, black bean, or white bean. For the chili, use turkey or ground beef.

Snack: 100 calories or less

Meal 3

Choose one of the following:

•1½ cups whole grain spaghetti with all, some, or none of the following (diced zucchini, squash, peppers, tomatoes, broccoli) in a marina or lemon-wine sauce)

•1 serving of 4 different vegetables

Snack: 100 calories or less

EXERCISE

•30 minutes of cardio/resistance training

*Notice and stick to the sequence of meals, snacks, and drinks

Meal 1:

Choose one of the following:

•2 scrambled eggs with cheese and diced veggies

•One 12-oz fruit smoothie with 1 scoop of protein powder (300 calories or less)

•One 12-oz protein shake (300 calories or less)

•One 8-oz yogurt parfait (300 calories or less)

•One large fruit salad bowl

Snack 1 (100 calories or less)

Snack 2 (100 calories or less)

Water: 2 cups of water infused with citrus (lemon, lime, orange, or grapefruit)

Meal 2: This must be consumed at least 6 hours after you've eaten Meal 1. This is your last meal for the day, so choose wisely and if you get hungry before going to bed, drink water (spritzed with

citrus) or tea (with honey and lemon if you choose)

Choose one of the following:

•1½ cups of soup or chili (for the soup, eat lentil, black bean, or

white bean. For the chili, use turkey or ground beef.

•1 serving of 4 different vegetables and a cup of cooked white or

brown rice

•large green garden (optional: tomatoes, peppers, 1 hard-boiled

egg, ¼ cup chunked avocado) with 3 tbsp balsamic vinaigrette

EXERCISE

•30 minutes of cardio/resistance training

BURN MELT SHRED
DAY 3

Meal 1

Choose one of the following:

•2-egg omelet with diced veggies and 3 oz cheese

•12 oz fresh fruit smoothie with 1 scoop protein or protein shake (300 calories or less)

•Energy bowl: Combine in a bowl ½ cup diced chicken, ½ cup brown rice, ¼ cup cubed cucumber, ¼ cup halved cherry tomatoes, 2 thin avocado slices, 2 tablespoons balsamic vinaigrette.

Snack: 100 calories or less

Meal 2

Choose one of the following:

•Bean, vegetable, cheese enchilada on whole-grain tortilla

•1 veggie and hummus sandwich on 100% whole-grain or whole-wheat bread

•1½ cups of soup or chili (for the soup, eat lentil, black bean, or white bean. For the chili, use turkey or ground beef.

Snack: 100 calories or less

Meal 3

Choose one of the following:

•6-ounce piece of garlic lemon herb chicken with roasted vegetables and 1⁄2 cup potatoes

•1½ cups whole-wheat pasta with diced chicken or fish

•Grilled or baked pork chop with 2 servings of vegetables

•1½ cups Poke bowl with brown rice, avocado, edamame, cucumber (add 3 oz chicken, steak, or fish)

Snack: 100 calories or less

EXERCISE

•Rest Day

DAY 4

Meal 1

Choose one of the following:

•1 grilled cheese sandwich on 100% whole-grain or whole-wheat bread

•1 cup low-fat or nonfat plain Greek yogurt with ⅓ cup granola or muesli and ¼ cup berries

•One 12-oz fruit smoothie with 1 scoop of protein powder (300 calories or less)

•One 12-oz protein shake (300 calories or less)

Snack: 100 calories or less

Meal 2

Choose one of the following:

•Black bean wrap with avocados, diced tomatoes, lettuce, and brown rice on whole grain tortilla

•large garden green salad (optional: grapefruit, nuts, peppers, tomatoes, sunflower seeds)

Snack: 100 calories or less

Meal 3

Choose one of the following:

•1 saucy sloppy joe and a serving of vegetables or small green garden salad (see recipe in RECIPES chapter)

•6-oz grilled chicken or fish with ¾ cup brown rice (cooked) and one green vegetable

•4 servings of 4 different steamed or raw veggies and 1 cup cooked brown or white rice

•1½ cups whole grain spaghetti with all, some, or none of the following (diced zucchini, squash, peppers, tomatoes, broccoli) in a marina or lemon-wine sauce)

Snack: 100 calories or less

EXERCISE

•30 minutes of cardio/resistance training

*Notice and stick to the sequence of meals, snacks, and drinks

Meal 1

Choose one of the following:

•2 scrambled eggs with cheese and diced veggies

•One 12-oz fruit smoothie with 1 scoop of protein powder (300 calories or less)

•One 12-oz protein shake (300 calories or less)

•One 8-oz yogurt parfait (300 calories or less)

•One large fruit salad bowl

Snack 1 (100 calories or less)

Snack 2 (100 calories or less)

Water: 2 cups of water infused with citrus (lemon, lime, orange, or grapefruit)—consume these cups sometime between snack 2 and meal 2

Meal 2: This must be consumed at least 6 hours after you've eaten Meal 1. This is your last meal for the day, so choose wisely and if you get hungry before going to bed, drink water (spritzed with citrus) or tea (with honey and lemon if you choose)

Choose one of the following:

•1½ cups of soup or chili (for the soup, eat lentil, black bean, or white bean. For the chili, use turkey or ground beef.

•1 serving of 4 different vegetables and a cup of cooked white or brown rice

•large green garden (optional: tomatoes, peppers, 1 hard-boiled egg, ¼ cup chunked avocado) with 3 tbsp balsamic vinaigrette

EXERCISE

•30 minutes of cardio/resistance training

DAY 6

Meal 1

Choose one of the following:

•1 protein shake (300 calories or less, no sugar added)

•1 fruit smoothie with 1 scoop of protein powder (300 calories or less, no sugar added)

•One 8-oz yogurt parfait with granola and fresh fruit

•1 fruit platter (3 servings of fruit)

Snack 1: 100 calories or less

Meal 2

Choose one of the following:

•1½ cups of soup or chili (for the soup, eat lentil, black bean, or white bean. For the chili, use turkey or ground beef.

•4 servings of veggies (cooked or raw) with 1 cup cooked white or brown rice

•1 large green salad (optional: olives, 2 tbsp shredded cheese, 5 cherry tomatoes, 2 tbsp of nuts) with 2 tbsp of vinaigrette-type dressing

•1½ cups whole-wheat or whole-grain pasta in a marinara sauce with vegetables (squash, broccoli, tomatoes, etc.) and 3 oz chicken or fish optional

•1 large green salad with veggies, but no croutons or bacon bits (NO creamy salad dressing)

Snack 2: 100 calories or less

Meal 3

Choose one of the following:

•large green garden (optional: tomatoes, peppers, 1 hard-boiled egg, ¼ cup chunked avocado) with 3 tbsp balsamic vinaigrette and 3 oz of chicken or fish; if you choose the vegetarian/vegan route and don't want the chick or fish, please make sure you have a cup of beans in your salad

•1½ cups of soup or chili (for the soup, eat lentil, black bean, or white bean. For the chili, use turkey or ground beef.

•6 oz chicken or fish with cup beans and cup cooked white or brown rice

EXERCISE

•Rest Day

DAY 7

Meal 1

Choose one of the following:

•1½ cups of cold cereal (sugars should be 7 grams or less)

•2-egg omelet with diced veggies and 3 oz cheese

•1 protein shake (300 calories or less, no sugar added)

•1 fruit smoothie with 1 scoop of protein powder (300 calories or less, no sugar added)

Snack: 100 calories or less

Meal 2

Choose one of the following:

•2 slices of tomato-cheese toasts on 100% whole-grain or whole-wheat bread

•bean burrito with cheese and sour cream in whole grain flour tortilla (use black or refried beans, low sodium)

•1½ cups of soup or chili (for the soup, eat lentil, black bean, or white bean. For the chili, use turkey or ground beef.

•5 oz turkey, veggie, or beef burger with small green garden salad

Snack: 100 calories or less

Meal 3

Choose one of the following:

•vegetable stir-fry in olive oil with broccoli, brown rice, peppers, carrots, soy sauce, mushrooms honey

•1½ cups of soup or chili (for the soup, eat lentil, black bean, or white bean. For the chili, use turkey or ground beef)

•6 oz chicken, turkey, or fish with 2 servings of vegetables

Snack: 100 calories or less

EXERCISE

•40 minutes of cardio—break it up into a morning and afternoon/evening session

CHAPTER 8

Week 7

"It's not how fast you start the race rather how strong

you're able to finish."

GUIDELINES

♦Drink 1 cup of water before every meal! Do not take your first

bite until you have finished the entire cup.

♦Your first meal can't be eaten before 3 hours after getting up.

Your last meal must be completed BEFORE two hours of going to

sleep. So, if you go to sleep at 10 PM, your last meal must be

completed by 8 PM.

◆Do your workout before you eat your first meal (fasted workout). Make sure to hydrate before the workout. If you need some energy, you can have an 8 oz yogurt or piece of fruit 30 minutes before the workout

◆2 cups of coffee allowed each day (drink as cleanly as possible—don't load with creams and too much sugar and extra calories; use just a little)

◆Drink one cup of lemon water—hot or cold—each day. You choose the time.

◆If you are a vegan or vegetarian, you can, of course, eliminate the animal products and make substitutions accordingly. However, please try to eat as many high protein non-animal foods as possible when make the substitutions

◆For your second meal this week, make sure you eat and finish 2 hours before going to sleep.

◆Snacks must come from SNACKS chapter

◆This week there are certain days where you get a **Floating Bonus Snack**. This means you get an extra 100 calorie snack if you need it. This bonus snack is in addition to the other snacks already listed

for that day. You can have this bonus snack whenever you want

during that day. If you don't eat this snack, it doesn't mean you

can carry it over to another day. You either use it or lose it.

♦Organic or raw, unfiltered honey is allowed

♦Organic 100% Stevia is allowed

♦NO artificial sweeteners

♦NO Frying—except the stir-fry veggies in olive oil

♦NO white bread

♦NO soda

♦NO white pasta

♦1 serving alcohol allowed each day

Meal 1

•Must have 1 piece of fruit. (Choose from the following, though you can choose others; pear, apple, ½ cup of raspberries or strawberries or blueberries or blackberries, ½ grapefruit, ½ cup of cherries.)

Choose one of the following:

•2 pancakes the size of a CD with 1 strip of bacon and 1 tbsp of 100% maple syrup

•2 scrambled eggs (diced veggie and 1 tablespoon shredded cheese optional; little butter or cooking spray allowed)

•1 egg white omelet (2 egg whites or ½ cup Egg Beaters; diced veggies optional) 1 cup of oatmeal

•1 cup of cold cereal with milk (Make sure the cereal total sugar is less than 7g)

Beverages

•You can have 1 cup of fresh juice (not from concentrate) *or* 1 cup of low-fat, reduced fat, or fat free milk, or unsweetened soy or almond milk

•You can have 1 cup of coffee (50 calories or less) along with the juice or milk should you choose to drink them

Optional: unlimited plain water

Eat your snacks 90-100 minutes after your meal!

Snack 1: ½ cup roasted pumpkin seeds *or* 10 baked whole-wheat pita chips *or* any other item 150 calories or less

Snack 2: 1½ cups of puffed rice or 1 cup broccoli florets with 2 tablespoons of dip or any other item 100 calories or less

Snack 3: Any item 150 calories or less

Meal 2

Choose one of the following:

•6-ounce piece of chicken (baked or grilled, no skin, not fried) with 2 servings of vegetables

•6-ounce piece of turkey (baked or grilled, no skin, not fried) with 2 servings of vegetables

•6-ounce piece of fish (baked or grilled, not fried) with 2 servings of vegetables

Beverages

Choose one of the following. Regardless of your choice, you can have unlimited plain flat or fizzy water.

•1 cup of flavored water

•1 cup of lemonade (fresh only)

•1 cup unsweetened iced tea

•1 cup of juice (not from concentrate)

•1 cup of low-fat, reduced-fat, or fat-free milk or unsweetened soy or almond milk

Snack 4: 100 calories or less

EXERCISE

•40 minutes. Choose a combination of the items below to fulfill your exercise requirement:

Gym Options

☐ 15 minutes walking/running on treadmill

☐ 15 minutes on elliptical machine

☐ 15 minutes on stationary bicycle

☐ 15 minutes swimming laps

☐ 15 minutes on stair climber

☐ 15 minutes of spinning

☐ 15 minutes of rowing machine

☐ 20 minutes treadmill intervals

Non-Gym Options

☐ 5 sets of running high knees (35 seconds or running followed by 35 seconds of rest is equivalent to 1 set)

☐ 4 sets of stationary squats (15 squats per set)

☐ 15 minutes jogging outside

☐ 225 jump rope revolutions

☐ 15 minutes of brisk walking

BURN MELT SHRED

☐ 15 minutes of walking up and down a staircase of at least 10 stairs; walking up and down the staircase is considered to be 1 set (rest between sets as needed)

☐ 15 minutes of Zumba

☐ 15 minutes of riding bicycle outside

☐ 15-minute hike

☐ 15 minutes of any other high-intensity cardio

☐ 15 minutes alternating between running and walking. Run for 1 minute, then walk for 1 minute, then run again and walk again. Repeat the cycle for 15 minutes.

☐ 10 sets of jog punches (45 seconds active exercise, then 30 seconds rest equals 1 set)

Advanced (note that doing the below exercises as described below will fulfill 15 minute-exercise commitment, even if it doesn't take 15 minutes to complete them. In fact, in most cases, you can finish them in half that time depending on your level of conditioning and how aggressive you are.)

☐ 3 sets of jump squats (10 consecutive jumps per set)

☐5 sets of mountain climbers (30 seconds continuous exercise followed by 35 seconds of rest is considered to be one set)

☐3 sets of box jumps (10 consecutive jumps per set)

☐3 sets of tuck jumps (10 consecutive jumps per set)

☐5 sets of ice skaters (35 seconds of exercises followed by 35 seconds of rest is considered to be 1 set)

☐3 sets of jumping lunges (10 consecutive jumps per set)

Meal 1

•Must have 1 piece of fruit or ½ cup of berries

Choose one from the following:

•1 cup of cooked oatmeal

•1 cup of Cream of Wheat or Farina

•1 cup of cold cereal with milk (Makes surge the cereal has 7g of sugar or less)

•6-ounce low-fat or fat-free yogurt; add fresh fruit

Beverages

•You can have 1 cup of fresh juice (not from concentrate) *or* 1 cup of low-fat, reduced fat, or fat free milk, or unsweetened soy or almond milk

•You can have 1 cup of coffee (50 calories or less) along with the juice or milk should you choose to drink them

Optional: unlimited plain water

Snack 1: 6 Ritz crackers or ½ blueberry muffin or any snack item 150 calories or less

Snack 2: 10 baby carrots with 2 tablespoons of low-fat hummus or ½ frozen banana dipped in chocolate or any snack item 100 calories

Snack 3: Any snack item 150 calories or less

Meal 2

Choose one of the following:

•2 slices of small cheese pizza (no larger than 4 inches across the crust and 6 inches long) with 2 servings of vegetables

•1 serving of lasagna (with or without meat) 4 inches x 3 inches x 1inch

•1 veggie burger (3 inches in diameter, ½ inch thick) with 2 servings of vegetables

•6 ounces of turkey or chicken (grilled or baked, no skin, not fried) with 2 servings of vegetables

Beverages

BURN MELT SHRED

Choose one of the following. Regardless of your choice, you can have unlimited plain flat or fizzy water.

• 1 cup of flavored water

• 1 cup of lemonade (fresh only)

• 1 cup unsweetened iced tea

• 1 cup of juice (not from concentrate)

• 1 cup of low-fat, reduced-fat, or fat-free milk or unsweetened soy or almond milk

Snack 4: 2 ounces of smoked salmon or 6 oysters or any snack item 100 calories or less

EXERCISE

• 30 minutes. Choose 2 of the following exercises for a total of 40 minutes:

Gym Options

☐ 15 minutes walking/running on treadmill

☐ 15 minutes on elliptical machine

☐ 15 minutes on stationary bicycle

☐ 15 minutes swimming laps

☐ 15 minutes on stair climber

☐ 15 minutes of spinning

☐ 15 minutes of rowing machine

☐ 20 minutes treadmill intervals

Non-Gym Options

☐ 5 sets of running high knees (35 seconds or running followed by 35 seconds of rest is equivalent to 1 set)

☐ 4 sets of stationary squats (15 squats per set)

☐ 15 minutes jogging outside

☐ 225 jump rope revolutions

☐ 15 minutes of brisk walking

☐ 15 minutes of walking up and down a staircase of at least 10 stairs; walking up and down the staircase is considered to be 1 set (rest between sets as needed)

BURN MELT SHRED

☐ 15 minutes of Zumba

☐ 15 minutes of riding bicycle outside

☐ 15-minute hike

☐ 15 minutes of any other high-intensity cardio

☐ 15 minutes alternating between running and walking. Run for 1 minute, then walk for 1 minute, then run again and walk again. Repeat the cycle for 15 minutes.

☐ 10 sets of jog punches (45 seconds active exercise, then 30 seconds rest equals 1 set)

Advanced (note that doing the below exercises as described below will fulfill 15 minute-exercise commitment, even if it doesn't take 15 minutes to complete them. In fact, in most cases, you can finish them in half that time depending on your level of conditioning and how aggressive you are.)

☐ 3 sets of jump squats (10 consecutive jumps per set)

☐ 5 sets of mountain climbers (30 seconds continuous exercise followed by 35 seconds of rest is considered to be one set)

☐3 sets of box jumps (10 consecutive jumps per set)

☐3 sets of tuck jumps (10 consecutive jumps per set)

☐5 sets of ice skaters (35 seconds of exercises followed by 35 seconds of rest is considered to be 1 set)

☐3 sets of jumping lunges (10 consecutive jumps per set)

Note: Don't forget that you're allowed a **Floating Bonus Snack** today!

Meal 1

•1 piece of fruit or ½ cup of berries

Choose one of the following. Make sure its 200 calories or less; no sugar added.

•1 fruit smoothie

•1 protein shake

Beverages

•You can have one cup of fresh juice or cup of coffee that's 50 calories or less.

•You can have unlimited plain water, flat or fizzy

Snack 1: 1 cup of grape tomatoes or ½ cup roasted chickpeas or any other item 100 calories or less

Snack 2: Hardboiled egg with ½ cup sugar snap peas or ½ cup fat-free yogurt and ½ cup blueberries or any other item 100 calories or less

Snack 2: 1 medium cucumber sprinkled with balsamic vinaigrette or 9 *or* 10 black olives or any other item 100 calories or less

Meal 2: 1 cup of soup (no potatoes, no heavy cream). Good choices are chicken noodle, vegetable, lentil, chickpea, split pea, black bean, tomato basil, minestrone. Always be careful of sodium content! Must be 200 calories or less.

•½ cup of brown rice

•1 serving vegetables

Beverages

Choose one of the following.

•Unlimited plain water (flat or fizzy)

•1 cup of flavored water

•1 cup of lemonade (fresh only)

•1 cup unsweetened iced tea

EXERCISE

•Rest Day

DAY 4

Meal 1

•One 12-oz fruit smoothie

•One 12-oz protein shake for breakfast

Meal 2

•1½ cups of soup

Meal 3:

•1 large green salad with veggies, but no croutons or bacon bits (NO creamy salad dressing)

Meal 4:

•1½ cups of soup

3 snacks from the following list:

•1 piece of fruit

•20 raw almonds

•15 cashews

•25 dry roasted peanuts

•2 tablespoons of sunflower or pumpkin seeds

•1 medium banana and 1 tbsp cottage cheese

•2 stalks celery and 2 ounces hummus

•8 baby carrot sticks (or 20 cucumber slices) and 2 ounces of hummus

•1 small baked sweet potato with 2 tablespoons fat-free sour cream or a little butter

•2 cups of air-popped popcorn with small amount of salt

•1 fat-free chocolate or vanilla pudding

•1½ cups of sugar snap peas

•1 hardboiled egg (lightly salt and pepper to taste)

•15 olives

•1 cup of mixed raw vegetables with 1 tablespoon of balsamic vinaigrette

EXERCISE

•Rest Day: However, if you want to push yourself, 9,000 steps.

DAY 5

Meal 1

Choose one from the following:

•1 cup of cooked oatmeal with fruit, brown sugar, and milk optional

•1 cup of Cream of Wheat or Farina with fruit, brown sugar, and milk optional

•1 cup of cold cereal with milk with a piece of fruit or ½ cup berries

Beverages

•You can have 1 cup of fresh juice (not from concentrate) *or* 1 cup of low-fat, reduced fat, or fat free milk, or unsweetened soy or almond milk

•You can have 1 cup of coffee (50 calories or less) along with the juice or milk should you choose to drink them

Optional: unlimited plain water

Snack 1: 2 Fudgsicles or 1 small baked potato topped with salsa or any other item 150 calories or less.

Snack 2: Any item 150 calories or less

Snack 3: Any item 150 calories or less

Meal 2

Choose one of the following.

•1 cup of soup (no potatoes, no heavy cream). Good choices are chicken noodle, vegetable, lentil, chickpea, split pea, black bean, tomato basil, minestrone. Always be careful of sodium content!

•large green garden (optional: tomatoes, peppers, 1 hard-boiled egg, ¼ cup chunked avocado) with 3 tbsp balsamic vinaigrette (add 3 oz of chicken or fish if desired)

•1½ cups Poke bowl with brown rice, avocado, edamame, cucumber

Beverages

Choose one of the following.

•1½ cups Poke bowl with brown rice, avocado, edamame, cucumber

•Unlimited plain water (flat or fizzy)

•1 cup of flavored water

•1 cup of lemonade (fresh only) 1 cup unsweetened iced tea

•1 cup of juice (not from concentrate)

•1 cup of low-fat, reduced-fat, or fat-free milk or unsweetened soy or almond milk

Meal 3

•1 large green garden salad with 2 ½ ounces of sliced chicken (3 cups of greens). You may include a few olives, shredded carrots, and ½ sliced tomato or 5 grape tomatoes. Only 3 tablespoons of fat-free dressing, no bacon bits, no croutons.

Beverages

Choose one of the following. Try to choose a different beverage from the one you chose in meal 2.

•Unlimited plain water (flat or fizzy) 1 cup of flavored water

•1 cup of lemonade (fresh only)

•1 cup unsweetened iced tea

•1 cup of juice (not from concentrate)

•1 cup of low-fat, reduced-fat, or fat-free milk or unsweetened soy

or almond milk

Snack 4: 1 small scoop of low-fat frozen yogurt or 3 tablespoons

of all-natural granola or any other item 100 calories or less.

EXERCISE

•30 minutes of cardio of your choice. You can break this up into 2

sessions of 15-minute length

•12,000 steps (outside of the cardio sessions)

DAY 6 (Low-calorie day)

Note: Don't forget that you're allowed a **Floating Bonus Snack** today!

Meal 1

Choose one of the following.

•1 fruit smoothie (200 calories or less, no sugar added)

•1 protein shake (200 calories or less, no sugar added) and 1 piece of fruit

Beverages

Optional; unlimited plain water

Optional:1 cup of coffee (no more than 1 packet sugar. 1 tablespoon milk or half and half)

Snack 1: 1 cup of grape tomatoes or 1 ½ cups of fruit salad or any snack item 150 calories or less

Snack 2: small shrimp with 3 tablespoons cocktail sauce or ½ cup of low-fat salsa with 10 tortilla chips or any snack item 100 calories or less

Snack 3: 4 chocolate chip cookies the size of a poker chip or ½ cup roasted chickpeas or any snack item 150 calories or less

Meal 2

Choose one of the following. Make sure it is different from yesterday's second meal

•6-ounce piece of chicken (baked or grilled, no skin, not fried) with 2 servings of vegetables

•6-ounce piece of turkey (no skin, not fried) with 2 servings of vegetables

•6-ounce piece of fish (baked or grilled, not fried) with 2 servings of vegetables

•1 large green garden salad with 2 ½ ounces of sliced chicken (3 cups of greens). You may include a few olives, shredded carrots, and ½ sliced tomato or 5 grape tomatoes. Only 3 tablespoons of fat-free dressing. No bacon bits, no croutons.

•1 cup of whole-grain pasta with marinara sauce (ground meat optional) with 2 servings of vegetables

•1 saucy sloppy joe and a serving of vegetables or small green garden salad (see recipe in RECIPES chapter)

Beverages

Choose one of the following.

•Unlimited plain water (flat or fizzy)

•1 cup of flavored water

•1 cup of lemonade (fresh only)

•1 cup unsweetened iced tea

•1 cup of juice (not from concentrate)

•1 cup of low-fat, reduced-fat, or fat-free milk or unsweetened soy or almond milk

Snack 4: Any item 100 calories or less

EXERCISE

•Rest Day

Meal 1

Choose one from the following:

•8-ounce yogurt parfait

•1 egg-white omelet (made with 2 egg whites or ½ cup of Egg Beaters; little butter or cooking spray is allowed

•1 cup of cold cereal with milk with one piece of fruit

Optional: 1 piece of 100 percent whole grain or whole wheat toast

Beverages

•You can have 1 cup of fresh juice (not from concentrate) *or* 1 cup of low-fat, reduced fat, or fat free milk, or unsweetened soy or almond milk

•You can have 1 cup of coffee (50 calories or less) along with the juice or milk should you choose to drink them

Optional: unlimited plain water

Snack 1: Any item 150 calories or less

Snack 2: 1 medium cucumber sprinkled with balsamic vinaigrette or 9 *or* 10 black olives or any other item 100 calories or less

Snack 3: Any item 150 calories or less

Meal 2

• 1 cup of brown rice

• 1 cup of cooked beans, chickpeas, or lentils (no baked beans)

• 1 serving of vegetables

Beverages

Choose one of the following. Regardless of your choice, you can have unlimited plain flat or fizzy water.

• 1 cup of flavored water

• 1 cup of lemonade (fresh only)

• 1 cup unsweetened iced tea

• 1 cup of juice (not from concentrate)

• 1 cup of low-fat, reduced-fat, or fat-free milk or unsweetened soy or almond milk

Snack 4: Any item 150 calories or less

EXERCISE

30 mins. Choose 2 of the following exercises for a total of 40 minutes:

Gym Options

☐15 minutes walking/running on treadmill

☐15 minutes on elliptical machine

☐15 minutes on stationary bicycle

☐15 minutes swimming laps

☐15 minutes on stair climber

☐15 minutes of spinning

☐15 minutes of rowing machine

☐20 minutes treadmill intervals

Non-Gym Options

☐5 sets of running high knees (35 seconds or running followed by 35 seconds of rest is equivalent to 1 set)

☐4 sets of stationary squats (15 squats per set)

☐15 minutes jogging outside

☐225 jump rope revolutions

☐15 minutes of brisk walking

☐15 minutes of walking up and down a staircase of at least 10 stairs; walking up and down the staircase is considered to be 1 set (rest between sets as needed)

☐15 minutes of Zumba

☐15 minutes of riding bicycle outside

☐15-minute hike

☐15 minutes of any other high-intensity cardio

☐15 minutes alternating between running and walking. Run for 1 minute, then walk for 1 minute, then run again and walk again. Repeat the cycle for 15 minutes.

☐10 sets of jog punches (45 seconds active exercise, then 30 seconds rest equals 1 set)

BURN MELT SHRED

Advanced (note that doing the below exercises as described below will fulfill 15 minute-exercise commitment, even if it doesn't take 15 minutes to complete them. In fact, in most cases, you can finish them in half that time depending on your level of conditioning and how aggressive you are.)

☐ 3 sets of jump squats (10 consecutive jumps per set)

☐ 5 sets of mountain climbers (30 seconds continuous exercise followed by 35 seconds of rest is considered to be one set)

☐ 3 sets of box jumps (10 consecutive jumps per set)

☐ 3 sets of tuck jumps (10 consecutive jumps per set)

☐ 5 sets of ice skaters (35 seconds of exercises followed by 35 seconds of rest is considered to be 1 set)

☐ 3 sets of jumping lunges (10 consecutive jumps per set)

CHAPTER 9

Week 8

"Life is one big road trip; how far you go isn't always in your control, but how much fun you have most certainly is. GO FULL BLAST!"

GUIDELINES

♦If you don't eat meat, make the substitutions appropriately with fish or vegetables.

♦3 alcoholic drinks allowed per week

♦Soups can be consumed with 2 saltine crackers if desired.

BURN MELT SHRED

♦For the regular, calorie days, you must consume 1 cup of water before eating a meal; you must consume 1 cup of water during your meal. You can add lemon or lime to your water, and you can drink fizzy water if you desire.

♦Be mindful of the three 500 calorie days that are in this week. Stick to it as closely as possible. Plan ahead!

♦You will be making a drink called the **Beat Back Drink** to help suppress your appetite between meals on the 500-calorie days. Here are the ingredients and instructions for the drink. This recipe makes 2 drinks, so save the other for later.

*2 cups of water (cold or warm)

*2 tbsp of fresh lemon juice

*1 tsp raw honey

*1 tsp crushed ginger root (dice or pulverize with mortar and pestle or food processor as fine as possible)

*1 tsp dried lavender

Bring warm water to a boil on the stove, then add honey, crushed ginger root, and dried lavender. Lower the temperature and let simmer for 3 minutes while stirring. Turn heat off and stir in the lemon juice. Divide into 2 cups. You can drink it warm or put it in the refrigerator and let chill and drink cold.

The **BEAT BACK** is an appetite suppressant drink that you must drink between meals 1 and 2.

♦You are allowed to drink coffee, but only 2 cups per day. Stay away from those fancy coffee preparations that add a lot of calories. Your coffee should contain no more than 100 calories

♦Don't eat your first meal until 2 hours after you are awake.

♦Do not eat the last meal within 2 hours of going to sleep. You can eat a 100-calorie snack before going to bed if desired.

♦Be smart in your snack choices. Avoid chips and doughnuts and candy; you can have them some of the time, but don't eat them often. They must fall within the calorie limit as described in the daily meal plan if you decide to have them, but please note these are not smart snacks nor beneficial to your long-term goals. If you must have something like these items, make it only one of your snacks for the day and use healthier options for the other snacks.

BURN MELT SHRED

♦You don't have to eat all of the food on the day's menu if you don't want to, but no skipping meals, no doubling up on meals, and no exceeding the meal guidelines in size and volume.

♦Condiments such as ketchup, mayo, and mustard are allowed, but no more than a teaspoon at each meal. The same goes for soy sauce.

♦You can consume unlimited spices

♦While fresh fruit is always preferred, canned and frozen fruit are allowed. Just make sure they are water-based and there are no added sugars.

♦Canned and frozen vegetables are allowed. Please be aware of the sodium content.

♦As far as beverages are concerned, you are allowed as much water as you like per day. Here are some other beverage guidelines:

♦Flavored waters allowed, but keep them under 60 calories

♦NO BREAD

♦NO SODA

♦NO FRIED FOOD

♦NO WHITE PASTA (except in the case of chicken noodle soup)

BURN MELT SHRED
DAY 1

Meal 1

Choose one of the following:

•1 small bowl of oatmeal (1.5 cups cooked) with 1 piece of fruit

•2 egg whites or I egg-white omelet with diced veggies (made with 2 egg whites max) with 1 piece of fruit

•1 small bowl of sugar-free cereal with fat-free, skim, or 1-percent fat milk with 1 piece of fruit

•One 8-ounce yogurt parfait with berries and ⅓ cup granola with 1 piece of fruit

Snack 1: 100 calories or less

Meal 2

Choose one of the following:

•1 large green garden salad with 3 oz of chicken or fish if desired. (Only 3 tablespoons of fat free dressing, no bacon bits, no croutons. Keep it clean.)

•1½ cups of soup (lentil, black bean, white bean, tomato, or cucumber)

•Chicken sandwich on 100% whole-wheat or whole grain bread with lettuce, tomato, 1 slice of cheese, and 1 tbsp of your preferred condiment

Snack 2: 150 calories or less

Meal 3

Choose one of the following:

•One 6-oz piece of grilled or baked chicken or fish with two servings of veggies

•1½ cups whole grain spaghetti with all, some, or none of the following (diced zucchini, squash, peppers, tomatoes, broccoli) in a marina or lemon-wine sauce)

•Portobello mushroom steaks (first marinade in spices and soy sauce or balsamic vinaigrette with a touch of olive oil to cook in and salt and pepper to taste)

Snack 3: 100 calories or less

EXERCISE

•Minimum 30 minutes. If you want to do more, all the better!

Work as hard as you can!

DAY 2 (500 Calorie Day)

*You are allowed to have 2 snacks today that total 150 calories together. You can break up the calories as you like. For example, each can be 75 calories. Or one might be 100 calories and the other might be 50. Whichever way you like.

Meal 1

•1 fruit smoothie or protein shake 150 calories

Beat Back Drink (1 cup)

Meal 2

•1 salad 125 calories

Beat Back Drink (1 cup)

Meal 3

•1 cup cooked brown or white rice with 2 serving of vegetables of your choice

EXERCISE

•Amount of exercise today: Minimum 30 minutes. If you want to do more, all the better! Work as hard as you can!

DAY 3

Meal 1

Choose one of the following:

•1 small bowl of oatmeal (1½ cups cooked) with 1 piece of fruit

•2 egg whites *or* 1 egg-white omelet with diced veggies (made with 2 egg whites max)

•1 small bowl of sugar-free cereal with fat-free, skim, or I-percent fat milk with 1 piece of fruit

•1 grilled cheese on 100-percent whole-grain or 100-percent whole-wheat bread with 1 piece of fruit

Snack: 150 calories or less

Meal 2

•1 large green salad w/3 tablespoons of vinaigrette dressing (options: 4 olives, 3 oz shredded cheese, 6 cherry tomatoes, ¼ cup nuts, ½ boiled egg; NO bacon, NO croutons, NO ham)

•Chicken salad on a bed of lettuce (toss 3-4 ounces shredded skinless roast chicken breast with ¼ cup sliced red grapes, 1 tbsp halved almonds, 1 tbsp plain, unsweetened Greek yogurt, and 1 tbsp mayonnaise.)

•4 servings of vegetables (Remember, a serving is about the size of the average person's fist.)

•Lettuce, cheese, tomato sandwich on 100% whole-grain or whole-wheat toast with your choice of spread

Snack: 150 calories or less

Meal 3

Choose one of the following:

•4 servings of vegetables, raw or cooked with 1 cup cooked brown or white rice

•6 oz grilled or baked chicken or fish with 2 servings of vegetables

•1 cup of whole grain pasta in a meatless tomato sauce with 1 serving of veggies mixed into the pasta

EXERCISE

•Rest Day

DAY 4 (500 Calorie Day)

*You are allowed to have 2 snacks today that total 150 calories together. You can break up the calories as you like. For example, each can be 75 calories. Or one might be 100 calories and the other might be 50. Whichever way you like.

Meal 1

•1 fruit smoothie or protein shake 150 calories

Beat Back Drink (1 cup)

Meal 2

•1 salad 125 calories

Beat Back Drink (1 cup)

Meal 3

•1 cup cooked brown or white rice with 2 serving of vegetables of your choice

EXERCISE

•Rest Day

DAY 5

Meal 1

Choose one of the following:

•6 ounces of low fat, plain yogurt; add sliced fresh fruit

•1 egg-white omelet (made with 2 egg whites or ½ cup of Egg Beaters; little butter or cooking spray is allowed

•1 cup of cold cereal or oatmeal with milk and 1 serving of fruit

•1 large fruit plate (½ sliced apple, ½ sliced grapefruit, 3 slices melon)

•**Optional:** 1 piece of 100 percent whole grain or whole wheat toast

Snack: 150 calories or less

Meal 2

Choose one of the following:

•4 servings of cooked or raw vegetables

•1½ cups of soup (options: black bean, white bean, tomato, gazpacho, lentil, chickpeas, vegetable, squash, pea); NO creamy or potato soups

Snack: 150 calories or less

Meal 3

Choose one of the following:

•4 servings of vegetables, raw or cooked

•One 6-oz piece of grilled or baked chicken or fish with two servings of veggies

•1 large green salad w/3 tablespoons of vinaigrette dressing (options: 4 olives, 3 oz shredded cheese, 6 cherry tomatoes, ¼ cup nuts, ½ boiled egg; NO bacon, NO croutons, NO ham)

EXERCISE

•Minimum 30 minutes. If you want to do more, all the better! Work as hard as you can!

DAY 6 (500 Calorie Day)

*You are allowed to have 2 snacks today that total 150 calories together. You can break up the calories as you like. For example, each can be 75 calories. Or one might be 100 calories and the other might be 50. Whichever way you like.

Meal 1

•1 fruit smoothie or protein shake 150 calories

Beat Back Drink (1 cup)

Meal 2

•1 salad 125 calories

Beat Back Drink (1 cup)

Meal 3

•1 cup cooked brown or white rice with 2 serving of vegetables of your choice

EXERCISE

•Rest Day

DAY 7

Meal 1

Choose one of the following:

• 2 pancakes the size of a CD with 2 strips of bacon (turkey)

• 2 scrambled eggs (diced veggie and 1 tablespoon shredded cheese optional; little butter or cooking spray allowed)

• 1 egg white omelet (2 egg whites or ½ cup Egg Beaters; diced veggies optional) 1 cup of oatmeal

• 1 cup of cold cereal

Snack: 150 calories or less

Meal 2

• 2 small slices of cheese pizza with small green garden salad

• 1 large green salad w/3 tablespoons of vinaigrette dressing (options: 4 olives, 3 oz shredded cheese, 6 cherry tomatoes, ¼ cup nuts, ½ boiled egg; NO bacon, NO croutons, NO ham)

•1 bowl of soup (no potatoes, no cream). Good choices are chicken noodle, vegetable, lentil, chickpea, split pea, black bean, tomato bisque, etc. Be careful of sodium content with 1 serving of veggies

•1 veggie and hummus sandwich on 100% whole-grain or whole-wheat bread

•burrito bowl—1½ cups—brown rice, beans of your choice, tomato, avocado, onion, shredded lettuce

Snack: 150 calories or less

Meal 3

Choose one of the following:

•1 large green salad w/3 tablespoons of low-fat vinaigrette dressing (options: 4 olives, 3 oz shredded cheese, 6 cherry tomatoes, ¼ cup nuts, ½ boiled egg; NO bacon, NO croutons, NO ham) with 3 oz of diced chicken or fish

•6-ounce piece of chicken (no skin, no frying) with 2 servings of vegetables

•6-ounce piece of fish (no frying) with 2 servings of vegetables

•6-ounce piece of turkey (no skin, no frying) with 2 servings of vegetables

•4 servings of vegetables with 1 cup cooked or brown rice

•1 saucy sloppy joe and a serving of vegetables or small green garden salad (see recipe in RECIPES chapter)

EXERCISE

•40 minutes of cardio broken up into 2 sessions—one in the morning, the other in the afternoon

CHAPTER 10

BURN MELT SHRED

RECIPES

Breakfast Energy Bowl

Pumpkin Oatmeal

Egg Whites and Herbs Wraps

Gramma's "Won't She Do It!" Pancakes

Boston's Delicious Green Monster

Banana Oatmeal Breakfast

Georgia's Sweetest Peach

Mad Blue Mango

Butter Lettuce Salad Supreme

Bean, Cucumber, and Tomato Ensemble

Tongue Lickin' Turkey Chili

Tomato Dunked Black Bean Soup

Hearty Spinach Soup

Tender Baked Sea Bass

Spicy Grilled Chicken

Protein-Packed Salmon Pasta

Vegetarian Sweet Potato Pesto Pasta

Saucy Sloppy Joes

Cheesy Stuffed Pork Chops

Splendiferous Wedge Salad

BREAKFAST ENERGY BOWL

Serves: 1

One 5.3-ounce container plain nonfat Greek yogurt

½ teaspoon honey

Pinch ground cinnamon

2 tablespoons rolled oats

Zest of 1 lemon

1 tablespoon dried blueberries

1 teaspoon roasted unsalted sunflower seeds

In a small bowl, combine the yogurt, honey, cinnamon, oats, and lemon zest and stir to mix. Let stand about 5 minutes to soften the oats. Sprinkle the blueberries and sunflower seeds over the top and enjoy.

BURN MELT SHRED
PUMPKIN OATMEAL

Serves: 4

1 cup low-fat milk

½ teaspoon cinnamon

Pinch ground cloves

Pinch salt

¼ cup canned puréed pumpkin

2 tablespoons honey

2 cups old-fashioned rolled oats

1/3 cup chopped toasted pecans

½ teaspoon pure vanilla extract

1. In a large saucepan over medium heat, combine the milk, 1 ½ cups water, cinnamon, cloves, and salt, and bring to a boil.

2. Whisk in the pumpkin and honey until incorporated. Stir in the oats and pecans and simmer, stirring frequently, until the oats are just cooked, 2 to 3 minutes.

3. Remove the pan from the heat, stir in the vanilla extract, and let stand for a few minutes before serving.

EGG WHITES AND HERBS WRAPS

Serves: 2

2 large egg whites

1 tablespoon low-fat milk

1 tablespoon chopped flat-leaf parsley

½ tablespoon chopped fresh chives

3 large basil leaves, finely chopped

½ tablespoon unsalted butter

Two 8-inch whole-wheat tortillas, warmed

¼ cup shredded reduced fat mozzarella cheese

1. In a medium bowl, combine the egg whites and milk and whisk until frothy and foamy. Add the parsley, chives, and basil and whisk again.

2. Melt the butter in a large nonstick skillet over medium-low heat, swirling to coat the pan. 3. Add the eggs and cook, stirring slowly with a rubber spatula, until the eggs are set, about 5 minutes.

4. Divide the eggs among the tortillas and sprinkle about 1 tablespoon of the cheese over the eggs on each tortilla. Wrap the tortillas, folding in the ends like a burrito.

5. Serve immediately or wrap in aluminum foil to keep warm until ready to eat.

GRAMMA'S "WON'T SHE DO IT!" PANCAKES

Serves: 4

1 egg

1½ cups all-purpose flour

1¼ cups whole milk

½ teaspoon pure vanilla extract

3 teaspoons baking powder

1 tablespoon granulated sugar

½ teaspoon salt

2 tablespoons unsalted butter, melted, plus more as needed

(optional)

Cooking spray

1. In a large bowl, sift together the flour, baking powder, sugar, and salt.

2. Make a well in the center of the dry ingredients and pour in the milk, vanilla extract, butter, and egg. Stir just until mixed and the batter is free of lumps. Let the batter rest for 5 minutes.

3. Coat a large skillet with cooking spray and heat it over medium heat (or heat the skillet over medium heat and add a small amount of melted butter). Pour about ¼ cup of batter into the skillet for each pancake. Cook until golden brown on the underside and then flip. Continue cooking until both sides are brown and serve warm.

BOSTON'S DELICIOUS GREEN MONSTER

Serves: 2

Less than 200 calories

1 cup kale

1 medium cucumber, peeled and sliced

1 large green apple, peeled, cored, and sliced

1 teaspoon fresh grated ginger

1½ tablespoons fresh lemon juice

1 tablespoon honey

10 ice cubes

Place all ingredients except the ice and blend for 1 minute. Add the ice and honey and purée until smooth and creamy. This recipe makes multiple servings; drink only one at this time.

BANANA OATMEAL BREAKFAST

Serves: 1

Less than 200 calories

½ cup fat-free plain or vanilla yogurt

⅓ cup oatmeal

⅓ cup low-fat or fat-free cow's milk (soy, almond, and oat milk

can be substituted)

¼ banana, peeled and sliced

½ teaspoon honey

½ cup crushed ice

Combine all ingredients in a blender and purée until smooth.

GEORGIA'S SWEETEST PEACH

Serves: 2

Less than 200 calories

2 large peaches, pitted and sliced (or ¾ cup of frozen peach slices)

2 cups fresh or frozen strawberries

4 tablespoons fat-free plain or vanilla yogurt

6 ice cubes

2 teaspoons honey (optional)

Combine all ingredients in a blender and purée until smooth. This recipe makes multiple servings; drink only one at a time.

Ian K. Smith, MD
MAD BLUE MANGO

Serves: 1

Less than 200 calories

½ cup sliced mango

½ cup blueberries

½ cup fat-free plain or vanilla yogurt

1 small banana, peeled and sliced

¼ cup milk

½ teaspoon honey (optional)

Combine all ingredients in a blender and purée until smooth. This recipe makes multiple servings; drink only one at this time.

BUTTER LETTUCE SALAD SUPREME

Serves: 4

1 large head butter lettuce, torn into bite sized pieces

2 navel oranges, peeled

¼ cup pitted Kalamata olives, chopped

⅓ cup sliced almonds, toasted

1 tablespoon white wine vinegar

½ teaspoon whole-grain Dijon mustard

2 teaspoons chopped fresh tarragon

2 teaspoons finely minced shallot

2 tablespoons extra-virgin olive oil

Salt and freshly ground black pepper, to taste

Spread the lettuce on a serving platter. Divide each orange in half using the segments as a guide. Slice the orange halves crosswise into half-moon slices and arrange them on top of the lettuce. Scatter the olives and almonds over the salad.

In a small bowl, whisk together the vinegar, mustard, tarragon, and

shallot until combined. Add the olive oil, season with salt and

pepper as needed, and whisk until thick and emulsified.

Drizzle the dressing over the salad and serve.

BURN MELT SHRED
BEAN, CUCUMBER, AND TOMATO ENSEMBLE

Serves: 4

2 cups green beans, trimmed

1 cup kidney beans

1 cup chopped cucumbers

¼ cup red wine vinegar

4 tablespoons extra-virgin olive oil, plus more for drizzling

Juice of 1 large lemon

Juice of ½ lime

3 medium heirloom tomatoes, cut into wedges

1 pint cherry tomatoes, halved lengthwise

Kosher salt and freshly ground black pepper, to taste

Bring a medium pot of water to a boil; cook green and kidney beans for 3-4 minutes, not to long where they are no longer crunchy. Drain beans and spread on paper towels to dry. Whisk vinegar, olive oil, lime and lemon juice, salt, and pepper in a bowl until combined. Transfer beans to tray or platter and add the cucumbers evenly throughout. Drizzle with dressing. Salt, and

pepper.

TONGUE LICKIN' TURKEY CHILI

Serves: 6 to 8

2 tablespoons extra-virgin olive oil

1 pound lean ground turkey

1 yellow onion, chopped

3 cloves garlic, chopped

1 yellow bell pepper, chopped

1 tablespoon tomato paste or tomato puree

1 tablespoon chili powder

One 14-ounce can organic crushed tomatoes

2 cups water mixed with 2 tablespoons extra-virgin olive oil

One 15-ounce can reduced-sodium cannellini beans, rinsed and drained

One 15-ounce can reduced-sodium kidney beans, rinsed and drained

One 15-ounce can reduced-sodium pinto beans, rinsed and drained

Freshly ground black pepper to taste

Sliced scallions for serving

1. Heat oil in a large saucepan over medium heat. Add turkey and break it up with a wooden spoon. Cook until browned, 6 to 8 minutes. Add onion, garlic, and bell pepper and cook, stirring, until softened, 6 to 8 minutes.

2. Add tomato paste and chili powder and cook, stirring, until the paste begins to caramelize, 3 to 4 minutes.

3. Bring to a simmer and cook until liquid has reduced by half, about 5 minutes. Add tomatoes, water with oil in it, and beans. Bring to a boil.

4. Reduce the heat to a simmer, cover, and cook until very thick, 35 to 40 minutes. Season with black pepper to taste. Garnish with the scallions and serve.

BURN MELT SHRED
TOMATO DUNKED BLACK BEAN SOUP

Serves: 6

Less than 200 calories

1 tablespoon olive oil

1 medium onion, peeled and diced

One 15-ounce can kidney beans

One 15-ounce can black beans

2 medium tomatoes, diced

1 green bell pepper, diced

½ teaspoon garlic powder

1 cup low-sodium chicken stock

3 cups water

3 tablespoons fresh lemon juice

In a small pot or saucepan, sauté onions in olive oil until tender, 5 to 7 minutes. Combine onions with other ingredients in a large pot. Cover and cook on medium heat for 10 minutes, stirring occasionally, then reduce heat and simmer for 10 minutes.

HEARTY SPINACH SOUP

Serves: 4

Less than 200 calories

1 teaspoon olive oil

½ medium onion, peeled and finely chopped

2 gloves garlic, peeled and minced

1 stalk celery, finely chopped

1 cup jasmine rice

2 cups low-sodium vegetable chicken broth

1 cup of water

1 six-ounce bag of baby spinach

1½ cups low-fat or fat-free milk Salt and pepper

In a large pot or saucepan sauté onions and garlic in olive oil over medium heat, 5 to 7 minutes. Add chicken broth, water, rice, and celery to the garlic and onions. Bring to a boil, cover, and simmer for 10 minutes. Stir in the spinach, reduce heat, cover and simmer until leaves are nice and tender, 5 minutes. Reduce heat and add milk. Let simmer for 3 to 5 minutes. Add everything into blender or food processor and purée until creamy. Salt and pepper to taste.

TENDER BAKED SEA BASS

Serves 2

2 cloves garlic, minced

1 tablespoon Italian seasoning

1 tablespoon extra-virgin olive oil

1 teaspoon ground black pepper

1 teaspoon sea salt

⅓ cup white wine vinegar

Two 6-ounce sea bass fillets (cleaned and scaled)

2 lemon wedges

1. Preheat oven to 450 degrees.

2. In a small bowl, mix garlic, Italian seasoning, oil, parsley, pepper, and salt.

3. Place fish in baking pan and rub mixture on both sides of fish evenly, then pour vinegar over fish.

4. Bake for 10 to 15 minutes, until fish flakes.

5. Pour vinegar over fish.

6. Bake fish for 15 to 20 minutes, until fish flakes.

7. Serve hot with lemon wedges.

Ian K. Smith, MD
SPICY GRILLED CHICKEN

Serves 4

1 teaspoon garlic powder

1 teaspoon ground cumin

½ teaspoon ground coriander

3 tablespoons olive oil

½ teaspoon sea salt

¼ teaspoon ground black pepper

4 chicken breasts

1. Preheat oven to 400 degrees.

2. In a small bowl, mix garlic powder, cumin, coriander, oil, salt, and pepper.

3. Use a basting brush to rub mixture over both sides of chicken.

4. Place chicken on a broiler pan and bake on each side for about 5 minutes, depending on the thickness of the breast. Make sure to cook all the way through so that there's no pink in the middle.

5. Serve hot.

BURN MELT SHRED
PROTEIN-PACKED SALMON PASTA

Serves 4

1 pound whole-wheat penne or rigatoni pasta

Sea salt and freshly ground black pepper to taste

One 1-pound salmon fillet

½ cup fresh basil leaves, finely chopped

2 teaspoons capers

2 cloves garlic, minced

Grated zest and juice of 1 lemon

2 tablespoons extra-virgin olive oil

½ teaspoon red pepper flakes

1 teaspoon freshly grated Parmesan cheese

1. Preheat oven to 375 degrees.

2. Cook pasta in a large pot of boiling salted water, until al dente.
Drain well.

3. Season salmon with salt and pepper to taste, then place on a parchment paper–lined baking pan and bake for 15 to 20 minutes, until desired temperature is reached.

4. In a large bowl, toss pasta with basil, capers, garlic, lemon zest, lemon juice, oil, red pepper flakes, and salt and pepper to taste.

5. Cut salmon into bite-size pieces. Add it to the pasta bowl and gently toss, making sure not to break up the salmon pieces.

6. Serve hot, topped with parmesan.

VEGETARIAN SWEET POTATO PESTO PASTA

Serves: 4

1 cup frozen shelled edamame, thawed

2 cloves garlic, chopped

¼ cup sliced almonds, toasted

¼ cup fresh flat-leaf parsley leaves

Grated zest of ½ lemon

½ cup freshly grated parmesan cheese, plus more for garnish

¼ cup extra-virgin olive oil, plus more as needed

Sea salt and freshly ground black pepper to taste

1 pound whole-wheat spaghetti or penne pasta

2 sweet potatoes, cut into ¾-inch cubes

30 green beans, trimmed and cut in half

1. To make pesto sauce, combine edamame, garlic, and almonds in the bowl of a food processor and pulse until finely chopped. Add parsley, lemon zest, parmesan, and oil and pulse until well

combined and the edamame is very finely chopped. Transfer pesto to a large mixing bowl and season with salt and pepper.

2. Bring a large pot of water to a boil with a pinch of salt, then boil pasta, sweet potatoes, and green beans until pasta is al dente and potato and green beans are very tender—about 10 minutes. Drain, and reserve 4 tablespoons of the cooking water, setting it aside.

3. Transfer pasta, potato, and green beans to a large bowl. Stir in pesto and cooking water and toss well until the sauce is a creamy texture. Season to taste. Divide among plates, drizzle with oil, and serve.

BURN MELT SHRED
SAUCY SLOPPY JOES

Serves: 6-8

One 14.5-ounce can reduced-sodium diced tomatoes

1 cup organic ketchup (for lower sodium option, use no-salt ketchup)

½ tablespoon Worcestershire sauce

½ tablespoon Dijon or brown mustard

1 teaspoon red wine vinegar

2 tablespoons pure maple syrup

1 tablespoon chili powder

1½ teaspoon cumin

1½ pounds lean ground turkey

2 teaspoons olive oil

1 large carrot, finely diced

2 cup finely diced red, yellow, or orange bell pepper

1 medium yellow onion finely diced

2 cloves garlic, minced

8 whole-wheat hamburger buns, toasted

1. In a medium bowl, combine the tomatoes, ketchup, Worcestershire sauce, mustard, vinegar, maple syrup, chili powder, and cumin. Whisk the sauce to combine and set aside.

2. In a large skillet over medium-high heat, brown the ground turkey. Drain well and transfer the turkey to a bowl. Set aside.

3. Heat the olive oil in a large skillet over medium heat. Add the carrot and sauté until soft. Add the bell peppers and onion and cook until soft and translucent. Add the garlic and sauté until fragrant, about 1 to 2 minutes.

4. Reduce the temperature to low and add the sauce. Simmer for 10 minutes, stirring frequently. Add the ground turkey, stir to combine, and simmer for 5 minutes or until warmed through.

5. Spoon the mixture onto the toasted hamburger buns

CHEESY STUFFED PORK CHOPS

Serves: 4

4 boneless pork loin chops, about 1 inch

½ cup marinated artichokes, drained, liquid reserved

12 whole-wheat crackers (about 1-inch square), crushed

1 ounce Swiss cheese, finely diced

Salt and freshly ground black pepper, to taste

½ tablespoon extra-virgin olive oil

1½ cups cooked brown rice, for serving

1. Preheat oven to 400 degrees F.

2. Use a sharp, thin knife to slice the pork chops in half horizontally without slicing all the way through.

3. In the bowl of a food processor, pulse the artichokes until they are finely chopped, then transfer them to a large bowl. Add the cracker crumbs and cheese. Drizzle enough of the artichoke marinade over the stuffing to moisten it.

4. Open the pocket you cut in each pork chop, and fill with the stuffing. Skewer the pockets with toothpicks to close them. Season both sides of the chops with salt and peppers.

5. Heat the olive oil in a large, ovenproof, nonstick skillet over medium-high heat. Add the pork chops and cook until browned, 3 to 4 minutes. Flip the chops and transfer the pan to the oven.

6. Cook until bottoms of the chops are golden and the chops are completely cooked through, 10 to 12 minutes. Remove from the oven and remove the toothpicks. Serve with cooked rice.

SPLENDIFEROUS WEDGE SALAD

Serves: 4

½ cup low-fat buttermilk

2 tablespoons chopped fresh chives, plus more for garnish

2 tablespoons chopped fresh flat-leafed parsley

⅓ cup nonfat plain yogurt

½ teaspoon salt

Freshly ground black pepper to taste

1 small clove garlic, chopped

1 small head iceberg lettuce, cut into 4 wedges

½ cup cherry or grape tomatoes, halved

Chopped fresh chives, for garnish

1. Combine the yogurt, buttermilk, chives, parsley, salt, pepper, and garlic in the container of a small food processor or blender and purée until smooth.

2. Place the lettuce wedges on 4 salad plates. Drizzle the dressing

evenly over the wedges. Top each wedge with a scattering of

tomatoes and fresh chives and serve.

CHAPTER 11

BURN MELT SHRED

SNACKS

100 Calories or Less

Fruits

• ½ small apple, sliced, with 2 teaspoons peanut butter

• ¼ cup loosely packed raisins

• 1 cup mixed berries (try raspberries, blueberries, or blackberries)

•Citrus-berry salad: 1 cup mixed berries (raspberries, strawberries, blueberries, and blackberries) tossed with 1 tablespoon freshly squeezed orange juice

•2 medium kiwis

•¼ avocado, smashed, on a whole-grain cracker, sprinkled with balsamic vinegar and sea salt

•Stuffed figs: 2 small, dried figs stuffed with 1 tablespoon reduced-fat ricotta and sprinkled with cinnamon

•1 cup cherries

•30 grapes

•1 cup strawberries

•2 small peaches

•3 pineapple rings in natural juices

•2 cups watermelon chunks

•3 dried apricots stuffed with 1 tablespoon crumbled blue cheese

BURN MELT SHRED

•Small baked apple (about the size of a tennis ball) dusted with cinnamon

•Chocolate banana: ½ frozen banana dipped in two squares of melted dark chocolate

•2 pineapple rounds, each ¼ inch thick, grilled or sautéed

•5 frozen yogurt-dipped strawberries (dip strawberries in yogurt, then freeze)

•1 medium grapefruit sprinkled with ½ teaspoon sugar, broiled if desired

•6 dried apricots

•4 dates

•3 fresh figs

•½ pound fruit salad

•1 pomegranate

•1 nectarine

•3 to 4 tablespoons dried cherries

•1 fat-free mozzarella cheese stick with ½ medium apple (about the size of a baseball), sliced with skin left on

•1 cup fresh red raspberries with 2 tablespoons plain yogurt

•½ cup diced cantaloupe topped with ½ cup low-fat cottage cheese

Veggies

•Kale chips: ⅔ cup raw kale (stems removed) baked with 1 teaspoon olive oil at 400°F until crisp

•½ medium baked potato with a touch of butter or 1 tablespoon sour cream

•1 medium red pepper, sliced, with 2 tablespoons soft goat cheese

•10 baby carrots with 2 tablespoons hummus

•5 cucumber slices topped with ⅓ cup cottage cheese and salt and pepper

•White bean salad: ⅓ cup white beans, a squeeze of lemon juice, ¼ cup diced tomatoes, 4 cucumber slices

BURN MELT SHRED

• ⅓ cup wasabi peas

• ½ cucumber (seeded) stuffed with one thin slice of lean turkey and mustard or fat-free mayonnaise

• Chickpea salad: ¼ cup chickpeas with 1 tablespoon sliced scallions, a squeeze of lemon juice, and ¼ cup diced tomatoes

• 1 ounce cheddar cheese with 4 to 5 radishes

• 1 ounce cream cheese with 4 to 5 celery sticks

• 2 stalks celery

• 3 oven-baked potato wedges

• 1 large carrot, raw

• ¾ cup carrots, cooked

• 1 cup broccoli florets with 2 tablespoons hummus

• ⅔ cup sugar snap peas and 3 tablespoons hummus

• ½ cup edamame and sea salt to taste

• 1 medium cucumber

• 1 cup lettuce, drizzled with 2 tablespoons fat-free dressing

•Greek tomatoes: 1 tomato (about the size of a tennis ball) chopped and mixed with 1 tablespoon feta cheese and a squeeze of lemon juice

•Cheesy breaded tomatoes: 2 roasted plum tomatoes, sliced and topped with 2 tablespoons breadcrumbs and a sprinkle of organic Parmesan cheese

•1 cup sliced zucchini, seasoned with salt to taste

•Grilled portobello mushroom stuffed with roast veggies and 1 teaspoon shredded low-fat cheese

•1 cup radishes, sliced or chopped

•1 medium ear of corn on the cob with seasoning

•1 medium tomato with a pinch of salt

•⅓ cup canned red kidney beans

•1 medium tomato, sliced, with a sprinkle of feta cheese and olive oil

•1 baked medium tomato sprinkled with 2 teaspoons organic Parmesan cheese

•Black bean salsa over 3 roasted eggplant slices

•3 medium breadsticks with hummus

•1 tablespoon peanuts and 2 tablespoons dried cranberries

•1 cup grape tomatoes

•¼ red bell pepper, sliced, ¼ cup thin carrot slices, ¼ cup guacamole

•½ cup black beans topped with 2 tablespoons guacamole

•Stuffed tomatoes: 10 halved grape tomatoes stuffed with a mixture of ¼ cup low-fat ricotta cheese, 1 tablespoon diced black olives, and a pinch of black pepper

Nuts and Seeds

•10 cashews

•2 tablespoons sunflower seeds

•17 pecans

•2 tablespoons poppy seeds

•2 tablespoons pumpkin seeds

•2 tablespoons flaxseeds

•25 peanuts, oil-roasted

•3 tablespoons roasted unsalted soy nuts

•12 chocolate-covered almonds

•½ cup roasted pumpkin seeds (keep in shells)

Dairy

•½ cup low-fat or fat-free plain Greek yogurt with a dash of cinnamon and 1 teaspoon honey

•1 small scoop low-fat frozen yogurt

•1 strip low-fat string cheese

•¾ ounce sharp cheddar cheese cubes

•4 to 6 ounces fat-free or low-fat plain Greek yogurt

•½ cup low-fat cottage cheese with ¼ cup fresh pineapple slices

BURN MELT SHRED

On the Go

•Leaf lettuce roll-up stuffed with a single slice of ham or beef and cabbage, carrots, or peppers

•Tropical cottage cheese: ½ cup fat-free cottage cheese with ½ cup chopped fresh mango and pineapple

•1 hard-boiled egg with everything bagel seasoning

•8–10 chocolate kisses

•½ cup fat-free yogurt and ½ cup blueberries

•½ whole-wheat English muffin topped with 1 teaspoon fruit butter

•6-ounce glass of orange juice (try making frozen juice pops for a cooling treat)

•2 slices of deli turkey breast

•Watermelon salad: 1 cup raw spinach with ⅔ cup diced watermelon, sprinkled with 1 tablespoon balsamic vinegar

•Strawberry salad: 1 cup raw spinach with ½ cup sliced strawberries and 1 tablespoon balsamic vinegar

•Crunchy kale salad: 1 cup kale leaves, chopped, with 1 teaspoon honey and 1 tablespoon balsamic vinegar

•Cucumber sandwich: ½ English muffin with 2 tablespoons cottage cheese and 3 slices cucumber

•Cucumber salad: 1 large cucumber, sliced, with 2 tablespoons chopped red onion and 2 tablespoons apple cider vinegar

•1 hard-boiled egg and ½ cup sugar snap peas

•Turkey roll-ups: 4 slices smoked turkey rolled up and dipped in 2 teaspoons honey mustard

•½ cup unsweetened applesauce with 1 slice of 100% whole-wheat toast, cut into 4 strips for dunking

•9 to 10 black olives

•½ cup raisin bran

•1 cup grape tomatoes and 6 wheat crackers

•7 saltines

BURN MELT SHRED

•Spicy black beans: ¼ cup black beans with 1 tablespoon salsa and

1 tablespoon fat-free Greek yogurt

•⅔ ounce dark chocolate

•Mini rice cakes with 2 tablespoons low-fat cottage cheese

•One 11½-ounce can low-sodium V8 100% vegetable juice

•½ sheet matzo

•20 grapes with 15 peanuts

•⅓ cup cooked quinoa

•¼ cup low-fat granola

•½ cup oat cereal, toasted

•½ cup clam chowder, preferably tomato-based

•5 pitted dates stuffed with 5 whole almonds

•½ cup unsweetened applesauce mixed with 10 pecan halves

Meat and Seafood

•6 large clams

•3 ounces cooked fresh crab

•1½ ounces cooked Pacific halibut

•2 ounces cooked lobster

•10 cooked bay scallops

•4 cooked large sea scallops

•2 ounces cooked yellowfin tuna

•8 small shrimp and 3 tablespoons cocktail sauce

•2 ounces smoked salmon

•6 oysters

•10 cooked mussels

•3 ounces tuna, canned in water

•½ cup canned crab

•3 ounces cooked cod

•2 ounces lean roast beef

BURN MELT SHRED

Fun

•15 mini pretzel sticks with 2 tablespoons fat-free cream cheese

•25 oyster crackers

•6 saltine crackers with 2 teaspoons peanut butter

•4 whole-wheat crackers and 2 servings fat-free cheese

•Guac and chips (5 tortilla chips and ⅓ cup guacamole)

•1 thin brown-rice cake spread with 1 tablespoon peanut butter

•Dark chocolate and peanut butter (½-ounce dark chocolate square with 2 teaspoons organic peanut butter)

•3 teaspoons natural peanut butter

•1 rice cake with 1 tablespoon guacamole

•3 crackers lightly spread with peanut butter

•About 40 goldfish crackers

•7 animal crackers

•3 cups air-popped popcorn

•2 cups air-popped popcorn with 1 teaspoon butter

•11 blue-corn tortilla chips

•1½ cups puffed rice

•½ cup low-fat salsa and 5 small (bite-size) tortilla chips

•2 graham cracker squares and 1 teaspoon peanut butter, sprinkled with cinnamon

•1 seven-grain Belgian waffle

150 Calories or Less

Fruit

•1 medium orange, sliced and topped with 2 tablespoons chopped walnuts

•15 frozen banana slices

•1 medium mango

•¾ cup halved strawberries topped with a squirt of whipped cream

BURN MELT SHRED

• ½ cup dried apricots

• 1 medium papaya with a squeeze of lime juice on top, sprinkle of chili powder optional

• 6 dried figs

• 25 frozen red seedless grapes

• 1 cup raspberries topped with a squirt of whipped cream

• 20 medium-size cherries

• 1 large apple, sliced, sprinkled with cinnamon

• 1 medium apple, sliced, with 1 tablespoon natural peanut butter spread on the slices

• 1 medium pear and 1 cup low-fat or skim milk

• ½ avocado topped with diced tomatoes and a pinch of pepper

• 1 cup blueberries with a squirt of whipped cream

Veggies

• ¾ cup roasted cauliflower with a pinch of sea salt

•10 baby carrots dipped in 2 tablespoons light salad dressing

•¾ cup steamed edamame (baby soybeans in the pods)

•½ medium avocado sprinkled with sea salt

•1 small baked potato topped with a mixture of salsa and 1 tablespoon shredded low-fat cheddar cheese

•1 cup sugar snap peas with 3 tablespoons hummus

•Loaded pepper slices: 1 cup red bell pepper slices topped with ¼ cup warmed black beans and 1 tablespoon guacamole

•Small baked potato topped with salsa

•1 medium red bell pepper, sliced, with ¼ cup guacamole

•Tasty pepper: 1 sliced bell pepper, marinated in 1 tablespoon balsamic vinegar, salt, and pepper

•½ cup roasted chickpeas

•1 cup grape tomatoes

•2 dill pickle spears

Nuts and Seeds

•9 chocolate-covered almonds

•½ cup shelled pistachios

•½ cup roasted pumpkin seeds, lightly salted to taste

•16 cashews

•21 raw almonds

•46 pistachios

•2 medium-size nectarines

Dairy

•½ cup low-fat cottage cheese with 1 tablespoon natural peanut butter mixed in

•1 chocolate fudge sugar-free pudding with 5 slices strawberries and a squirt of whipped cream

•1 slice of Swiss cheese and 8 olives

•1½ strips of low-fat string cheese

•2 scoops of sorbet

•1 small chocolate pudding

•½ cup light natural vanilla ice cream

•1 cup yogurt parfait and 1 tablespoon granola

•½ cup no-salt-added cottage cheese and almond butter

•1% cottage cheese mixed with 1 tablespoon almond butter

On the Go

•4 saltine jelly sandwiches: sugar-free jelly between 2 saltine crackers; 8 crackers in all

•Peanut butter and jelly: ½ whole-grain English muffin, 1 tablespoon peanut butter, and sugar-free jelly

•Egg salad: 2 whole eggs, ½ teaspoon low-fat mayo, and spices to taste spread on ½ toasted whole-wheat or whole-grain bagel

•16 saltines

BURN MELT SHRED

•Hummus and cucumbers: ½ large cucumber, chopped and combined with 2 tablespoons hummus

•Applesauce and cereal: 1 applesauce pouch and ½ cup dry cereal

•2 hard-boiled eggs with a pinch of salt and pepper

•2 frozen fruit bars (no sugar added)

•10 walnut halves and 1 sliced kiwi

•Baby burrito: 6-inch corn tortilla, 2 tablespoons bean dip, and 2 tablespoons salsa

•Kiwi and oats: 1 kiwi, sliced, with ½ cup oat cereal

•½ cup natural apple chips (no sugar or preservatives added)

•2 tablespoons hummus spread on 4 crackers

•1 cup grapes with 10 almonds

•Chocolate-dipped pretzels: Melt semisweet chocolate morsels in a microwave; dip 3 honey pretzel sticks in chocolate; put pretzels in freezer until chocolate sets.

•50 goldfish crackers

•Brown rice vegetable sushi rolls, 5 pieces

•1 cup sugar snap peas with 3 tablespoons low-fat hummus

•1½ cups fresh fruit salad

•¼ cup yogurt-covered raisins

•2 stalks celery and 2 tablespoons natural peanut butter

•Watermelon treat: 1 cup diced watermelon topped with 2 tablespoons crumbled feta cheese

•1 cup Cheerios

•6 watermelon skewers: 1 cube watermelon, 1 small cube feta cheese, and 1 slice cucumber on each of 6 toothpicks

•6 cucumber, cherry tomato, mozzarella ball skewers

•Mediterranean salad: 1 tomato, 1 medium cucumber, ½ diced red onion, sprinkled with 2 tablespoons low-fat feta cheese

•1 packet of plain instant oatmeal, ½ cup fresh blueberries, sprinkle of cinnamon

Meat and Seafood

•4 turkey slices and 1 medium apple, sliced

•1 can water-packed tuna, drained and seasoned to taste

•4 ounces chicken breast wrapped in lettuce and topped with dill
mustard

•Turkey wrap: 2 slices of deli turkey breast, whole-grain flatbread,
sliced tomatoes and cucumbers, and lettuce

•Turkey-wrapped avocado: ¼ avocado sliced into strips and
wrapped in 3 ounces deli turkey meat

•Tuna salad: One 5-ounce can water-packed light tuna, 1
tablespoon low-fat mayo, and 1 diced sweet pickle

Fun

•2 popsicles

•1 small banana, sliced, and ½ ounce dark chocolate

•2 ounces turkey jerky

•English muffin pizza: whole-wheat English muffin topped with 1 tablespoon tomato sauce, and 1 tablespoon organic Parmesan cheese and broiled

•2 squares graham cracker and 8 ounces skim milk

•4 chocolate-chip cookies, each a little larger than the size of a poker chip

•10 baked whole-wheat pita chips and 3 tablespoons salsa

•2 Fudgsicles

•Blueberries and sorbet: ½ cup fruit sorbet topped with ½ cup blueberries

•1 ounce of pretzels and 1 teaspoon honey mustard

•½ blueberry muffin

•1 cup strawberries dipped in 1 tablespoon melted semisweet chocolate chips

•12 small baked tortilla chips and ½ cup salsa

•7 olives stuffed with 1 tablespoon blue cheese

BURN MELT SHRED

•4 potstickers dipped in 2 teaspoons reduced-sodium soy sauce

•5 crackers lightly smeared with peanut butter

•2 cups air-popped popcorn sprinkled with 1 tablespoon organic

Parmesan cheese

FOLLOW Dr. Ian on Social

Instagram: @DoctorIanSmith

Twitter: @DrIanSmith

www.doctoriansmith.com

Facebook: @DrIanKSmith and

@BurnMeltShred

YOU CAN and MUST DO IT!

Made in the USA
Middletown, DE
20 January 2022

59164090R00146